Interferon and Cancer

Interferon and Cancer

Edited by
Karol Sikora
Ludwig Institute for Cancer Research
Cambridge, United Kingdom

Plenum Press • New York and London

Library of Congress Cataloging in Publication Data

Main entry under title:

Interferon and cancer.

Bibliography: p.
1. Interferon—Therapeutic use. 2. Cancer—Chemotherapy. I. Sikora, Karol.
[DNLM: 1. Interferons—Therapeutic use. 2. Interferons—Immunology. 3. Neoplasmas
—Drug therapy. QZ 267 I58]
RC271.I46I56 1983   616.99′4061   83-9626
ISBN 0-306-41379-5

© 1983 Plenum Press, New York
A Division of Plenum Publishing Corporation
233 Spring Street, New York, N.Y. 10013

Printed in the United States of America

PREFACE

Interferon was first discovered in 1957. Over the last five years it has become almost a household word. Many believe it to be a drug with already proven efficacy against cancer and viral infection. The media has distorted any cool scientific view of the data available. We have learned much about the complexity of the interferon system. We know some of the switches involved in interferon gene expression and its secretion by virally and immune stimulated cells. We also know that it binds to a cell surface receptor, mediating its complex effects on target cells by a series of second messengers. The advent of the new techniques of modern molecular biology, such as monoclonal antibodies and gene cloning, has had tremendous impact on the rate of acquisition of knowledge. Such techniques have provided us with almost unlimited quantities of highly purified interferon for clinical trial in patients with a spectrum of infectious and malignant diseases. The information we have gathered raises many more questions. Why should there be several families of interferon genes? What is their true physiological role? How are they interrelated functionally? Interferon is clearly a cellular hormone providing a means of communication between cells. Whether it has clinical value in the management of patients with diseased cells remains to be seen. This book summarises our current knowledge of interferons as possible anti-cancer agents. It is clear interferon is no penicillin for cancer. However it has been shown to have growth inhibitory effects for a variety of tumour types. By learning more about these effects previously hidden control mechanisms may be uncovered that we can exploit clinically.

Karol Sikora
Cambridge

v

CONTENTS

INTRODUCTION

KAROL SIKORA

Ludwig Institute for Cancer Research, MRC Centre
Hills Road, Cambridge

THE CANCER PROBLEM

One in five people in the Western world currently dies from
cancer. There are many organs in which cancer arises but it is the
common solid tumors that kill at least 90% of our cancer patients.
Over the last 20 years there has been a tremendous investment of
money and human resources to tackle the cancer problem. The United
States alone spends several billion dollars annually on cancer
research, both in the laboratory and clinic. If we consider the end
results in patients with common solid tumors then it is clear that
despite this enormous effort there is little to show in terms of
survival benefit. A sense of frustration has crept in amongst
researchers, clinicians, granting agencies, and ultimately the public
who must finance most cancer research.

The conventional methods for treating cancer are surgery,
radiotherapy, and chemotherapy. Surgery and radiotherapy can only be
effective in treating disease which has remained localized.
Metastases by definition cannot be encompassed in the treatment
fields. Chemotherapy is currently the only proven systemic therapy
available. There are several problems in using these treatments.
The first is measuring tumor load in an individual patient. Although
it is easy to observe a change in tumor size for some cancers, in
many patients it is difficult. An example is a patient who has an
excision of a breast cancer. Following surgery for the primary it is
difficult to assess if there are small deposits of metastatic disease
which require further therapy. Even patients with advanced disease
may pose assessment problems. In the patient with carcinoma of the
bronchus, for example, the size of an abnormality on a chest X-ray
may not necessarily represent tumor load. The pressure of the

1

carcinoma within the bronchus causes obstruction with resultant
collapse of lung segments giving rise to increased X-ray shadowing.
The change in size of the shadow therefore may not represent tumor
burden and its response to therapy. Another problem is the lack of
effective systemic therapies for these common tumors. The third
problem is the major one. We lack selectively toxic agents which can
destroy tumor cells, leaving their normal counterparts virtually
intact. Perhaps this is not so surprising. Tumor cells arise from
normal cells and share their biochemical processes. Normal cells
during certain phases of development behave very much like tumor
cells with periods of rapid growth, invasion, change in site and
motility: properties that in the fully differentiated tissue would
represent malignant change. There seems to be no specific
biochemical process unique to the malignant cell against which to
design our therapy. Any system in which there is a hint of selective
toxicity to tumor cells is of great interest to the clinical
oncologist.

It was against this backdrop that interferon made its entrance.
In the early 1960's its anti-tumor effects were observed _in vitro_ and
in animal studies. Serious clinical studies did not begin until the
1970's when adequate supplies were available. For the first time now
we have large amounts of interferon available to determine its true
place in the treatment of human cancer.

STRUCTURE

The complete purification and understanding of the structure of
the interferon has only recently been achieved. Even now there are
still details about which uncertainty exists (Rubinstein, 1982).
Standard biochemical techniques have allowed the separation of the
major families. The nomenclature is extremely confusing to the
newcomer in the field. It has grown up over the last 20 years as new
interferons have been discovered and new facts about them emerged.
There are three major families of human interferon; alpha, produced
by leukocytes; beta, produced by fibroblasts; and gamma, by
lymphocytes. Interferon was first purified by thiocyanate
precipitation and gel exclusion chromatography from these three
sources and used as an antigen to immunize animals. The antibodies
so produced were found to distinguish the different families of
interferon. A major problem is that different sources of interferon
do not necessarily produce IFN of one type. Stimulated leukocytes
produce both alpha and gamma IFN. Table I lists the essential
information to understand the nomeclature. Type I and type II
interferon could be distinguished by antibodies raised against
preparations that were thought to be pure. Stability at low pH is a
characteristic of leukocyte and fibroblast interferon but not that
produced by mitogen or antigen stimulated lymphocytes. There was
considerable confusion for some years as to whether to different

TABLE I

The Interferons

α	β	γ
leukocyte lymphoblastoid	fibroblast	immune
viral induced	viral induced	antigen) mitogen) induced
Type I	Type I	Type II
pH2 stable	pH2 stable	pH2 unstable
not glycosylated	glycosylated	glycosylated
at least 8 genes	at least 5 genes	single gene
no introns	introns (except β_1)	introns
on chromosome 9	dispersed on chromosomes 2,5,9	on chromosome 12

interferon types were glycosylated or not. It is now clear that alpha interferon is not (Allen and Fantes, 1980). Despite increasing sophistication of biochemical techniques such as electrophoresis, chromatography, and a variety of affinity columns techniques, it has only been the advent of gene cloning that has allowed the complete structural relationships of the interferons to be understood. It is also clear that there are more related molecules that have not yet been isolated. Their structure will no doubt be determined over the next few years.

GENE CLONING

It is the ability to isolate specific pieces of human DNA and expand them in unlimited quantities in bacteria that has enabled the rapid detailed analysis of the structure of interferon (Nagata et al., 1980; Goeddel et al., 1980). Leukocytes or cell lines are triggered into a high production state by a combination of Sendai virus and super-induction by metabolic inhibitors. The messenger RNA pool is extracted from these switched on cells. The RNA's coding for the interferons sediments at 12S. Differential centrifugation allows partial purification and enrichment for interferon mRNA (Berger et al., 1980). These mRNA's are used as templates for the production of cDNA (c for copy) by the enzyme, reverse transcriptase. The cDNA copies are inserted into plasmid vectors which are in turn replicated in bacteria. Of course many mRNA's are copied, not all of which code for interferon. The resulting cDNA library, however, can be amplified and maintained indefinitely. By a process of screening and elimination the interferon clones can be isolated. Once one sequence is found which codes for IFN, hybridization techniques can be used to identify other cDNA clones in the library which contain homologous sequences. DNA known to code for interferon can be labelled to a high specific activity with ^{32}P nucleotides. This labelled probe is now used to identify which clones in the library will hybridize to it (Goeddel et al., 1981). These clones are isolated and expanded and the relationship to the probe DNA ascertained. The technology has been made much simpler since the advent of rapid DNA sequencing techniques which enables large fragments of DNA to be sequenced precisely (Sanger, 1975).

INTERFERON GENES

The first cloning of interferon cDNA was reported in 1980. Two cDNA species designated IFN alpha-1 and IFN alpha-2 were then used to screen a total human DNA gene bank. At least 16 distinct genes have been found which cross-hybridize with the relevant probe. Human IFN-β has also been cloned and possibly five different sequences of the beta gene isolated (Taniguchi et al., 1980). IFN-γ DNA has also been isolated although only a unique chromosomal gene was found to correspond to it (Gray et al., 1982). The majority of studies have been with the alpha-interferon genes. These are transcribed into messenger RNA without any interruption of the reading sequence. No splicing step is required to produce mRNA ready for translation into protein. This indicates that there are no intervening sequences (introns) in the IFN-α DNA sequences. Both beta and gamma genes possess introns. The chromosomal location of these gene families has now been determined. The alpha family is closely linked and arranged in tandem on chromosome 9 (Owerbach et al., 1981). The data on chromosomal locations for beta and gamma genes is less clear cut. The new nomenclature of the recombinant era is outlined in Table II.

TABLE II

Interferons Available for Clinical Trial

Family	Species	Comment
Hu IFN α	Hu IFN α (PIF)	partially purified leukocyte
	Hu IFN α Leu	leukocyte
	Hu IFN α Lym	lymphoblastoid
	Hu IFN α N	Namalwa cell lymphoblastoid
	Hu rIFN α A	clone A recombinant*
	Hu rIFN α D	clone D recombinant*
	Hu rIFN α A/D	hybrid A/D recombinant*
	Hu rIFN α_2	clone α_2 (same as A)**
Hu IFN β	Hu rIFN β_1	β_1 clone recombinant
Hu IFN γ	Hu rIFN γ_1	γ_1 clone recombinant

*   Genentech – Hoffmann–La Roche
** Biogen – Schering Plough

CLINICAL TRIALS

The clinical effects of human interferons have been investigated
mainly using the alpha-interferons. Until 1978 the only preparation
available was that from pooled buffy coat leukocyte produced by the
Finnish Red Cross in Helsinki (Cantell, 1977). In the mid-70's
Burrough's Welcome in London invested considerable resources to
obtaining lymphoblastoid interferon. This was produced by growing a
human lymphoblastoid line (Namalwa) in tissue culture and collecting
spent supernatants. There were many problems in the purification
from the supernatants until the advent of a monoclonal antibody that
could be used on affinity columns. Human interferon-β has been
manufactured for clinical trial both from human diploid fibroblasts
and also from tumor cell lines. The first interferons produced by
recombinant techniques which were produced in industrial quantity
were both alpha. There are problems of nomenclature in that the
first to be cloned, human IFN α_2, is probably identical to human IFN
αA. Both of these are now available in large quantities in a highly
purified form. It is clear that in assessing any clinical trial the
quality of the product and its likely contaminants is of vital
significance. There are many products of lymphoid cells which may
affect the course of patients with cancer or infectious disease.
Until recently, clinical information on the use of interferon has

been scanty. It has been confined to a small series of patients who
are highly selected in terms of the disease studied.

INFECTIOUS DISEASES

Rational therapy for viral disease was clearly a main driving
force in the early days of clinical interferon research despite
inadequate supplies. The first demonstration of a positive effect in
man was its protection of volunteers against subsequent challenge by
influenza and rhino-viruses. Interferon was given as an intra-nasal
spray and the symptoms of viral infection were reduced, provided
treatment was given prior to viral infection. Whether prophylaxis
against upper respiratory tract infections can become a reality by
the use of exogenous interferon administration remains to be seen.
There are several serious acute viral infections in which interferon
has now been tried, including rabies, fulminating hepatitis, herpes
encephalitis, and Lassa fever (Taylor-Papadimitriou and Balkwill,
1982). The numbers of patients involved in these studies has been
extremely small with no control group. At present no firm
conclusions can be made as to the role of IFN in the management of
these diseases. The major problem in patients with viral disease is
that by the time signs and symptoms develop the virus has already
caused widespread intracellular damage. It therefore seems over
optimistic to expect systemic therapy at this stage to halt the
pathology that has resulted. At best limitation of disease could
occur.

In chronic viral infections the position is different. There
are several disease states, such as chronic hepatitis, chronic
cytomegalovirus, herpes simplex and Epstein Barr virus infections
where some patients develop a long term symbiosis with a virus. At
certain phases in the viral life history clinical problems result due
to the interaction between virus and host. A small percentage of
patients that develop classical infectious hepatitis, for example, go
on to develop chronic active hepatitis. In this latter disease the
virus persists in the liver causing continued degeneration of liver
parenchyma with a resulting cirrhosis. Virus particles persist in
the blood and are reduced or completely cleared by the administration
of interferon. Many adults harbor cytomegalovirus. In patients that
are immunosuppressed, cytomegalovirus can be a major problem causing
life threatening illnesses. Again interferon has been shown to
induce clinical and biological remissions in such patients.

NEUROLOGICAL DISEASES

Another category of diseases in which interferon has been used
in clinical trial is a hotchpotch of degenerative neurological
conditions. These include multiple sclerosis, motor neurone disease,

pre-senile dementia and subacute sclerosing panencephalitis (SSPE). These diseases have one feature in common - a poorly understood etiology. Claims of isolation of viruses have been made. Whilst convincing for SSPE, the evidence for a viral etiology of the other diseases is only circumstantial. A major problem in assessing the efficacy of any new therapeutic agent in these diseases is their natural periodicity. Periods of remission intertwine with periods of regression. There is also the profound psychological stimulus of any clinical trial. Only controlled studies can adequately assess the efficacy of the new drug in these distressing diseases.

CANCER

It is the anticancer potential of interferon that has led to the greatest recent interest in its clinical use. The early preparations of relatively impure interferon were shown to have some effect in causing objective tumor regression in patients with myeloma, breast cancer and non-Hodgkin's lymphoma (Sikora, 1980). However the responses tended to be partial rather than complete and transient in nature. The hope of pioneers in this field was that better tumor regression might be obtained if greater quantities of interferon were given to patients. The early preparations had serious side effects, principally fevers, malaise and fatigue. Because of the impurity of the interferons used at that time the question remained as to whether these effects were intrinsic to interferon or were a result of contaminants administered along with the interferon. The answers to these questions are beginning to emerge now that recombinant interferon of high purity is available for large scale clinical trials. The recombinant interferons also cause objective regression in certain tumor types and appear to be at least as biologically active as the naturally occurring preparation. As for toxicity, it is clear that pure interferon has profound side effects which limits the dose administered. Careful pharmacokinetic studies have shown that doses beyond 36 million units per day over periods of greater than one month are impossible to tolerate. Side effects at this dosage include anorexia, weight loss and central nervous system toxicity, which can present with features of a metabolic encephalopathy. All this makes the administration of interferon an arduous task for the clinical investigator.

Many trials are now in progress with interferon. So far tumor regression has only been observed consistently in patients with myeloma, non-Hodgkin's lymphoma and breast cancer. A small number of patients have now had well documented objective responses in diseases such as melanoma, renal cell carcinoma, lung cancer and Kaposi's sarcoma. The response rate in some of these tumors is low - less than 20%. It must be remembered however that the patients studied in these early phase II trials all have advanced disease, resistant to conventional therapy, and therefore any response whatsoever is encouraging indeed. Most of these responses have been partial, a reduction in tumor size rather than complete disappearance. There are many problems in assessing tumor load in an individual patient. It does seem likely however that most of these responses are real and that interferon is having a growth inhibitory effect on at least some tumors, either directly or through the immune system.

The outlook for patients with common solid tumors appears to have reached a plateau despite intense effort with conventional cytotoxic chemotherapy. With this background it seems reasonable to investigate further the anti-cancer potential of interferon. Now that adequate supplies are available there are many questions to address. If indeed it is working through an immuno-modulatory role then it might benefit patients with earlier disease in an adjuvant setting. Should it be given at the maximum tolerated dose or at a dose which has the greatest effect on the immune system? Despite the low response rate when used as a single agent in advanced disease, perhaps its combination with other systemic chemotherapy might provide beneficial results. How should it be scheduled in conjunction with other therapy?

It is clear that interferon is not to cancer what penicillin was to bacterial infection. However it may still have a part to play in the treatment of cancer patients. Only careful clinical and laboratory research in centers familiar with the rigors of such investigation can determine its eventual role in clinical oncology.

REFERENCES

Allen, G., and Fantes, K.H. 1980, A family of structural genes for human lymphoblastoid (leukocyte type) interferon, Nature, 287:408.

Berger, S.L., Hitchcock, M.J., Zoon, K.C., Birkenmeir, C., Friedman, R.M., and Chang, E.H. 1980, Characterisation of interferon messenger RNA synthesis in Namalva cells, J. Biol. Chem., 255:2955.

Cantell, K., Hervonen, S., Molensen, K.E., et al. 1977, Human leucocyte interferon: production, purification and animal experiments in: "The Production and Use of Interferon for the Treatment of Virus Infections", C. Walomouth, ed., p.35, The Tissue Culture Annual, Baltimore.

Goeddel, D.V., Shepard, H.M., Yelverton, E., et al. 1980, Human leukocyte interferon produced by E. coli is biologically active, Nature, 287:411.

Goeddel, D.V., Leung, D.W., Dull, T.J., et al. 1981, The structure of eight distinct cloned human leukocyte interferon cDNA's, Nature, 290:20.

Gray, P.W., Leung, D.W., Pennica, D., et al. 1982, Expression of human immune interferon cDNA in E. coli and monkey cells, Nature, 295:503.

Nagata, S., Taira, H., Hall, A., et al. 1980, Synthesis with E. coli of a polypeptide with human leucocyte interferon activity, Nature, 284:316.

Owerbach, D., Rutter, W.J., Shows, T.B., Gray, P., Goeddel, D.V., and Lawn, R.M. 1981, Leucocyte and fibroblast interferon genes are located on human chromosome 9, Proc. Natl. Acad. Sci. USA, 78:3123.

Rubinstein, M. 1982, The structure of human interferons, Biochimica et Biophysica Acta., 695:5.

Sanger, F., and Coulson, A.R. 1975, A rapid method for determining sequences in DNA by primed synthesis with DNA polymerase, J. Mol. Biol., 94:441.

Sikora, K. 1980, Does interferon cure cancer? Br. Med. J., 281:855.

Taniguchi, T., Ohno, S., Fujii-Kuriyama, Y., and Muramatsu, M. 1980, The nucleotide sequence of human fibroblast interferon cDNA, Gene, 10:11.

Taylor-Papadimitriou, J., and Balkwill, F. 1982, Implications for clinical application of new developments in interferon research, Biochemica et Biophysica Acta., 695:49.

HISTORICAL BACKGROUND

DAVID TYRRELL

Clinical Research Centre, Division of Communicable
Diseases, Watford Road, Harrow, Middlesex, HA1 3UJ

The discovery of interferon was the result of persistent
curiosity about how one virus in or on a cell could interfere with
the growth of another and the imaginative follow-up of some
unexpected results. Virus interference was a popular subject of
research, but we all had preconceptions, and no one thought of a
molecule mediating interference. I remember how, using pieces of
chick chorioallantoic membrane in buffered saline, we showed that
chemical inhibitors of virus multiplication stopped the development
of interference by apparently "dead" virus, but like others we
interpreted the results in terms of an entirely intracellular process
or processes. Isaacs and Lindenmann using a similar experimental
method tried to show, using virus stuck to red cells, that nucleic
acid escaped from the virus and entered the host cell to produce this
interference; they produced no conclusive results but found
unexpectedly that treated host cells were producing a
virus-inhibiting substance. They called this new secretion
interferon. Other workers in other countries reported independently
that they had found antiviral cell products of this sort but somehow
because of his clear experimental results and his excited
determination to discover both what the substance was and how it
worked (Lindenmann, 1982), Isaacs' publications became the focus of a
growing number of laboratory studies. Mind you, it was not agreed at
first that the interferon phenomenon was real; there were many
critical views at first and I still recall hearing the gibe of
"misinterpreton". It is difficult in retrospect to recapture the
limited view, the expectations and the puzzlement of an earlier age.
It was baffling that IFN seemed so difficult to purify, it was
strange that it seemed so variable - apparent differences in the
properties of different preparations were put down to poor technique
and it seemed that many different inducers fired off the synthesis of

11

the same substance by a particular cell; it seemed to produce effects
only in cells from related species; when more general biochemical
effects were detected such as those on oxidative metabolism, they
turned out to be due to contaminants.

We expected to be able to apply interferon to antiviral therapy
even though we did not understand it very well. It seemed to act
against a range of viruses and to be non-toxic for human cells - a
repeat of the penicillin story - and it was frustrating that although
monkey kidney interferon produced effects in human skin challenged
with vaccinia it seemed to have no effect against common colds. Why
was this? Were respiratory tract cells insusceptible? Were we using
too little interferon? And so on. This confusion perhaps explains
why the early observations that suggested that IFN might have an
effect on the growth of tumor cells were discounted (Paucker et al.,
1962). For one thing our minds were oriented towards viruses and for
another the experiments could be challenged - I think many of us
considered that the results were due to contaminating material. Of
course, early work had shown that IFN would prevent tumors of birds
induced by Rous Sarcoma Virus, but in that case the effect was
clearly on the replication of the virus and there was no effect if
one waited until the tumor had been induced. Fortunately work
continued, and Gresser (1982) has recently recounted the way ideas
changed as the experimental results came along during the 1970's. It
was assumed at first that virus-induced tumors of mice would be
inhibited by interferon and this was shown to be true, provided that
one gave enough interferon and started soon after the virus was
given. But then, contrary to expectation it was found that tumors
not induced by viruses were also inhibited. Then it was assumed that
this would be because IFN directly impaired the division of the tumor
cell, yet the effect was shown to be mediated largely through the
host, though it was also apparent that the effect was greatest when
interferon came into direct contact with the tumor cells. Although
the early experiments were done with crude interferon they were well
controlled; for example, comparison animals were given similar
material to that given to treated animals, such as extracts of normal
mouse brain in experiments in which virus infected brain was the
source of interferon. Nevertheless these effects were only fully
accepted as due to interferon after similar effects had been obtained
using highly purified preparations.

As this was going on it was becoming clearer that IFN's had
effects on many cell functions apart from the rather mysterious
inhibition of virus growth. It could stimulate the expression of
transplantation antigens and could enhance immunity, including
delayed hypersensitivity - the type of immune response involved in
the rejection of transplants and probably also in host mediated
limitation of tumor growth. As so often happens people became more
willing to accept an unexpected observation as it began to "fit in"
with preconceptions or with other experimental results. So the idea

that IFN's might modify tumors became more readily accepted.
However, some tumor biologists believed that this had no relevance to
whether, if comparable amounts of interferon could ever be
administered to man, it would have any effect on malignant disease.
They pointed out that many of the experiments were done with
implanted and no spontaneous tumors; that the tumors were not
syngeneic with the host; that there were few experiments in which any
effect had been shown on a tumor that had already developed, and so
on. It is probable that the experiments on patients with osteogenic
sarcoma in Sweden had more impact than much of the animal work. They
were only possible because of the pioneering work in Finland by
Cantell and his colleagues who developed methods of producing large
amounts of interferon from the white cells in the buffy coats of
blood donations from the Finnish Red Cross, and then of purifying it
sufficiently for clinical use. Patients were given standard primary
treatment, either amputation or local removal, and then a course of
daily interferon injections followed by maintenance therapy of three
injections a week. It became clear after a few years that patients
were having less pulmonary metastasis and were surviving longer than
those in a series of patients treated earlier in Sweden in the same
hospitals. The apparent benefits of IFN treatment were then
subjected to stringent criticism. Were the cases being given the
same primary treatments, and were they seen at the same stage of the
disease? Were the histological diagnoses acceptable? Because of the
views of clinicians it was not possible to have a randomized placebo
controlled trial, but a concurrent control group, managed without
interferon was recruited from other centers in Sweden, fully
realizing that this cannot control for minor local differences in the
management of cases.

A scientific training is a poor preparation for writing history
and a scientist is likely to produce nothing more than a dated list
of outstanding publications without indicating the forces in human
affairs that apparently determined how, when and where the scientific
advances occurred. I have already mentioned the names of outstanding
individual scientists who with their collaborators did key pieces of
laboratory work - Isaacs discovered interferon as an antiviral,
Gresser the antitumor activities and Cantell developed methods for
making human interferon. But these groups were extended by networks
of working visits and inter-laboratory collaborations. Baron and
Friedmann who were key workers in the USA spent time in Isaacs
laboratory. Gresser in France was interested in the effect of IFN on
tumor growth and collaborated with other nearby workers such as the
de Maeyers who were studying the biological and immunological effects
of IFN's and purifying mouse IFN. In Britain a formal committee was
set up between the Medical Research Council and three pharmaceutical
laboratories; Glaxo; ICI and Wellcome with the intention of quickly
applying interferon as an antiviral agent and protecting the process
of its manufacturing by taking out patents. It seems likely that the
guess that it would be a useful antiviral may well have been right

but the hopes of making it by a commercially viable process from
vertebrate cells were not really fulfilled - though after the
collaboration broke up the Wellcome Laboratories did produce good
interferon for clinical trials using suspended cultures of human
lymphoblastoid cells, as described elsewhere in this book.
Nevertheless, the committee played a valuable role in catalyzing
research. To me the most important result of its existence was that
we met at intervals, we discussed the field, assessed recent
publications, educated each other about what problems and
possibilities we could see from our point of view - biological,
chemical or clinical and we also co-operated practically, doing
together experiments we could not have done alone.

All the same, in spite of our systematic, directed and
co-ordinated research some of the most important events were
unforeseen. Two recent events of quite different sorts may be
mentioned. One is that clinical studies with inteferon were limited
to a few studies of antiviral activity, partly because of physical
lack of suitable interferon, which was limited largely to that made
in Helsinki, and also because of lack of finance. Then almost from
outside the scientific community there was sudden and really
premature enthusiasm for interferon as a cancer "cure". Lobbying and
meetings took place and particularly through the Amercian Cancer
Society and the National Cancer Institute funds became available to
finance the production of interferon from human white cells and
fibroblasts, and so more IFN was made and more trials were started.

However, the dramatic advance in understanding of the chemistry,
biology and molecular genetics of IFN's come as those developing the
subject of genetic manipulation saw IFN's as a suitable example on
which to demonstrate the possibility of gene cloning on an important
human molecule and providing a new supply of the substance from
genetically manipulated bacteria. Of course, in a sense, the
interferon field also contributed to that of genetic manipulation by
providing a basic corpus of biological facts, some sensitive
bioassays and fundamental physical and chemical information about the
molecules. Nevertheless we owe a great debt to the genetic
engineers.

The cynic says that the lesson of history is that no one learns
from history. Maybe it is naive to think that studying the history
of science makes us do better science. However, it may at least
enable us to understand better the science that is going on around
us. There is so much more to discover about interferon and cancer
that I think we should not be surprised if the course of research and
development shows many of the elements I have already described.
Certainly we should welcome and contribute bright new observations or
ideas on the biology of the field, we should encourage and take part
in multidisciplinary discussions and in practical research in the
area; much of the latter will probably be extensive and repetitive,

sorting true and general observations from the untrue and idiosyncratic. We should also be prepared for exciting new data, techniques or ideas to appear from time to time often from unforeseen events and to our great relief if we feel progress is slowing down. Writing history may be very difficult but we can, at least, all have a part in understanding and making it.

REFERENCES

Gresser, I. 1982, How does interferon inhibit tumour growth? <u>Phil. Trans. R. Soc. Lond. B</u>, in press.

Lindenmann, J. 1982, From interference to interferon: a brief historical introduction, <u>Phil. Trans. R. Soc. Lond. B</u>, in press.

Paucker, K. Cantell, K., and Henle, W. 1962, Quantitative studies on viral interference in suspended L cells. III Effect of interfering viruses and interferon on the growth rate of cells, <u>Virology</u>, 17:324.

METHODS OF PREPARATION

ARMIN H. RAMEL[*], W. COURTNEY McGREGOR[*] AND
ZOFIA E. DZIEWANOWSKA[+]

[*] Biopolymer Research Department, and [+] Department of
Medical Oncology and Immunology, Central Research
Division, Hoffmann-La Roche Inc., Nutley, N.J. 07110

INTRODUCTION

Assuming that the majority of readers will be clinical
investigators we tried to anticipate what such a specialist may
expect to find in this chapter. We concluded that a detailed
description of current methods of interferon preparation would not be
within the context of this book*. Rather than burden the reader with
technical details we decided to give an overview with emphasis on
advantages and disadvantages of current production methods and
present information about the origin, status of supply, and purity of
currently available interferon preparations. Aspects of product
quality we assumed would be of foremost importance. Such information
we believe will help in the planning of various clinical studies and
in the interpretation of results.

This chapter is undoubtedly written with a certain bias. We
have been party from the beginning to the scientific revolution of
recombinant DNA-technology and are associated with a leading
pharmaceutical company which has given major emphasis to this new
direction. The apparent miracle of modern molecular biology rapidly
unfolding before our eyes may produce a mirage of undue expectations.
The technology, however, is very real as are the products derived
from it.

----

* An up-to-date and detailed description of production and
purification methods is found in Methods in Enzymology, 78, S.
Pestka, eds., Academic Press, 1981.

Several therapeutically interesting proteins of high purity are now produced via recombinant DNA-technology in clinically significant amounts, including various interferons. Their production in kilogram amounts is now a matter of commitment only. In contrast to conventional tissue culture methods, recombinant DNA-technology holds the promise of practically unlimited supply once efficacy is proven in the clinic. Horowitz (1981) estimated that worldwide manufacturing capacity of leukocyte interferon from human white blood cells based on protocols developed by Cantell and coworkers (1981a; 1981b) exceeded 500 billion units in 1981 and that an additional amount of 12 trillion units could be mobilized within the voluntary blood banking community in this country alone. How do these numbers compare with the production capacity of recombinant DNA-technology? At a titer of 50 billion units per liter of bacterial fermentation broth - a level easily achieved by current methods - and a purification yield of 20%, it would require a single 50 liter fermentor operated 12 hours to produce the recombinant equivalent to the estimated 1981 supply of conventional interferon. In further contrast, the purity of the recombinant material from bacteria has been about 100 fold greater (>95% pure) than that of the product obtained from human cells (<1% pure).

In view of this extraordinary advantage of recombinant over conventional technology, one might be inclined to omit discussion of classic methods in a 1982 report on methods of preparation. This would be unrealistic since some clinical material continues to be produced by conventional technology. It would also be unfair in view of the pioneering efforts of Cantell and coworkers. Without their work on large-scale production, clinical studies with human leukocyte interferon could never have been initiated. Furthermore, many investigators have rightly questioned whether a single subtype of leukocyte interferon can substitute for the natural mix of subtypes and other interferons included in the body. Their natural distribution may depend on the type of tissue which is infected and the type of viral inducer. Further studies also may uncover synergistic effects between the subtypes and the various interferon classes (Fleischmann et al., 1979). Moreover, fibroblast and immune interferon are glycoproteins and it is not clear whether the carbohydrate moiety plays a role in their biological activity. Recombinant fibroblast interferon lacks carbohydrate and this will probably make any negative clinical results difficult to interpret. If sugar side chains are shown to be necessary for clinical efficacy with the fibroblast and/or immune interferons, then tissue culture methodology may continue to be important. On the other hand, methods are being developed which may provide in vitro glycosylation, if necessary, by means of enzymes.

Finally, we believe that the level of product purity arising from the various production methods will be a very important consideration for the reader. No material is ever 100% pure and the nature of the impurities as well as their relative concentration can be important. Impurities are of concern to the clinician for two main reasons: they may be antigenic and/or they may cause disturbing side effects. The impurities in preparations of recombinant interferons will obviously be of microbial origin. If administered over an extended period of time these impurities may give rise to antibodies. On the other hand antigenicity also may be inherent to those recombinant interferons which are sufficiently different from their natural counterpart, e.g. rIFN-beta. If registered by the body as a foreign substance they may elicit an immune response.

In summary, there are a number of reasons why interferons of natural origin may continue to be important. However, the potential problems enumerated for recombinant interferons may never materialize. Two of about 12 subtypes of recombinant leukocyte interferon already are in clinical trials. Others, including recombinant fibroblast and immune interferon, are expected to be available soon to be tested individually and in combination. Interferon cocktails of various compositions may well become powerful therapeutic weapons of the future.

PRODUCTION OF INTERFERONS BY TISSUE CULTURE TECHNOLOGY

With a few exceptions, interferon production in mammalian cells has to be induced by external stimuli. The most common viral inducers employed in large-scale interferon induction are paramyxo-viruses such as Newcastle disease and Sendai virus. The most common synthetic inducer is the double-stranded RNA polyrI·rC, formed by mixing of polyriboinosinic acid (polyrI) with polyribocytidylic acid (polyrC) in equimolar proportions.

The mechanisms of interferon production in the cell is very complex. The induction phase during which time the binding, uptake and processing of the inducer takes place can last from two to 16 hours dependent on the type of inducer. Induction by definition involves derepression of the interferon gene followed by transcrip-tion and translation of the interferon messenger RNA. In these instances where the interferon is glycosylated (e.g. beta interferon) postribosomal processing must follow translation.

A unique feature of interferon induction is a phenomenon called superinduction. Interferon production in cells which after induction are exposed to the metabolic inhibitors cycloheximide and actinomycin D (in that order) was found to be greatly increased. Ten to hundred times larger amounts of interferon are produced in superinduced vs. normally induced cells. Several other important phenomena related to the cellular control of interferon production have been discovered. Priming is one of them. If cells are pretreated with high-titer interferon before induction, an increased production of interferon is

observed. The knowledge of these biological features of interferon
production in the cell has greatly facilitated the development of
large-scale interferon production in tissue culture.

Three principle methods have emerged and are used for the
large-scale production of human alpha and beta interferon: (1)
stimulation by paramyxovirus of white blood cells from the buffy coat
of donated blood (2) stimulation by paramyxovirus of human
lymphoblastoid cells and (3) superinduction of human fibroblast
cultures with polyrI˙rC.

To date human gamma interferon has not been produced in
significant amounts. It is produced under special circumstances by
T-lymphocytes after stimulation with a mitogen or antigen (Epstein,
1981; Johnson et al., 1981). Work is in progress on the isolation
and purification of gamma interferon in many laboratories (O'Malley,
1981; Yip et al., 1981; Langford et al., 1979; Von Wussow et al.,
1982; de Ley et al., 1980).

Production with Normal Human Leukocytes

White blood cells from normal donors have been the chief source
of human leukocyte interferon employed in clinical or experimental
studies. Early studies by Gresser (1961) and Strander et al. (1966)
established that interferon production can be induced in normal human
leukocytes by paramyxoviruses. Sendai virus was found to be the most
effective. Newcastle disease virus instead of Sendai virus, however,
has been successfully used as inducer in various laboratories
(Waldman et al., 1981). This virus is sometimes preferred where
large volumes of Sendai virus constitute a potential hazard to local
mouse colonies. Leukocytes from patients with chronic myelogenous
leukemia have been used as a substitute for those from normal donors
by Herschberg et al. (1981). The classic induction and production
scheme developed by Cantell and coworkers is described in Methods in
Enzymology (1981).

White cells are either collected as buffy coats after whole
blood centrifugation or directly by leukapheresis. The washed
leukocytes are resuspended in a maintenance medium containing 'agamma
serum' and antibiotics to maintain sterility. Incubation is carried
out at 37.5°C in stirred ten to 20 liter carboys of suitable
construction. Priming as described above improves production of
interferon. Following induction with Sendai virus, cells and debris
are removed by either centrifugation or filtration. The supernatant
or filtrate contains the crude interferon at a concentration of 0.1
to 0.2 µg/ml, equivalent to about 8×10^4 IU/ml. The specific
activity of the crude interferon is about 6×10^4 to 8×10^4 IU/mg
protein and the purity at this stage is less than 0.1%.

Cantell et al. (1981b) and Horowitz (1981) have developed
protocols for large-scale partial purification based on potassium

thiocyanate and ethanol precipitation. Total recovery is about 90%
and the specific activity of the purified interferon ranges from 2.5
x 10^6 to 1.25 x 10^7 IU/mg protein.

Purification to homogeneity with specific activities up to 5 x
10^8 IU/mg has been accomplished by high-performance liquid
chromatography (Rubinstein and Pestka, 1981), by two-dimensional
polyacrylamide gel electrophoresis (Lin and Stewart, 1981), and by
immuno-affinity chromatography (Berg and Heron, 1981).

Production with Human Lymphoblastoid Cells

Human lymphoblastoid cell lines were first screened for
interferon production by Strander et al. (1975) and later by Johnston
et al. (1979). The line found most suitable for large-scale
production was the Namalva line established by Klein et al. in 1972.
Most lymphoblastoid cell lines are derived from Burkitt's lymphoma
and contain the human pathogen Epstein-Barr virus (EBV). DNA
-hybridization experiments, however, have shown that Namalva cells
contain only 50% of the EBV genome (Pritchett et al., 1976). The
possibility of accidental infection in work with these cells thus is
greatly reduced. Induction is achieved with paramyxoviruses
preferably with Sendai or Newcastle disease virus. About 80% to 90%
of the interferon induced by Sendai virus is of the alpha-type and
the rest (10% to 20%) is beta-type interferon (Havell et al., 1978).
Namalva cells can be grown to high cell density in suspension culture
in conventional tissue culture fermentors of practically any size.
Suspension cell culture is one of the most convenient and least
expensive ways to produce mammalian cell products such as interferon
on a large scale. Large-scale production of lymphoblastoid
interferon, hence, is actively pursued by many government
institutions and pharmaceutical companies around the world (Mizrahi,
1981; Bodo, 1981; Klein and Ricketts, 1981; Familletti et al., 1981a;
Zoon, 1981).

Namalva cells are grown in RPMI-1640 medium supplemented with
fetal bovine serum and various ingredients including antibiotics.
The seed culture used for the inoculation of the fermentors is
developed in a series of transfers. When cells have grown to the
appropriate cell density in the fermentor, cells are harvested,
resuspended in growth medium, and inoculated with the virus. Excess
virus is removed by centrifugation and cells are gently resuspended
in serum-free minimal medium. After incubation for 20 hours, cells
are removed by centrifugation and the supernatant is collected as
crude lymphoblastoid interferon. Titers achieved at this level range
from 1000 to 5000 IU/ml. Since the crude preparation contains very
low amounts of protein (40 to 80 µg/ml), specific activities of 2 x
10^4 to 7 x 10^4 IU/mg protein are routinely obtained. A large-scale
purification protocol which achieves roughly a 100-fold increase of
the specific activity has been reported by Bodo (1981) and

purification to homogeneity has been achieved by Zoon (1981). The
production of alpha-type interferon from a myeloblastoid cell lines
(KG-1 line) has been reported by Familletti et al. (1981a). The KG-1
cell line originated from a patient with acute myelogenous leukemia
(Koeffler and Golde, 1978). The interferon derived from this source
was purified to homogeneity by Hobbs et al. (1981).

Production with Normal Human Fibroblasts

Human diploid fibroblasts from foreskin or embryos are the third
major cell source for large-scale interferon production. Since these
cells can be carefully preselected, it is generally agreed that human
fibroblast interferon has the best safety potential in man. Large
stacks of cells can be built up easily so that supply of cells for
large-scale production is not a problem. Human fibroblasts are
anchorage-dependent and hence have to be grown as a monolayer
culture. Very promising systems which allow growth in suspension
tanks have recently been developed based on the use of micro-carriers
(Giard et al., 1979). These systems have a far better surface to
volume ratio than the conventional roller bottles.

For fibroblast interferon production confluent monolayer culture
of fibroblasts in roller bottles or multitray units are superinduced
as mentioned above. The culture medium (containing fetal bovine
serum and antibiotics) is removed and minimal essential medium (MEM)
containing polyI'rC and cycloheximide is added, followed after a
short incubation period by actinomycin D. The induction medium is
then replaced by a production medium (MEM containing 5% inactivated
human serum). After incubation for an additional 20 to 25 hours the
medium containing the interferon is harvested, pooled, and
centrifuged. The supernatant contains the crude fibroblast
interferon with titers ranging from 2.5 x 10^4 to 4 x 10^4 IU/ml and
specific activities from 5 x 10^4 to 1 x 10^5 IU/mg protein. In some
cell systems it has proven advantageous to include a priming step in
the induction protocol, i.e. to pretreat the cells for 24 hr with a
small amount of high-titer interferon prior to addition of the
inducer. Large-scale partial purification procedures achieving
specific activities of 2 x 10^7 IU/mg have been developed and reported
by Leong and Horoszewicz (1981) and by Van Damme and Billiau (1981).
Essentially homogeneous preparations with specific activities of up
to 5 x 10^8 IU/mg have been obtained by including one of the following
key steps in the purification protocol: affinity chromatography on
Blue Sepharose (Knight, 1981), high-performance liquid chromatography (Friesen et al., 1981; Kenny et al., 1981), or absorption on
controlled-pore glass followed by zinc-chelate chromatography (Heine
and Billiau, 1981).

A continuous fibroblastoid cell line (MG-63) derived from a
human osteosarcoma has been used successfully by Van Damme and
Billiau (Friesen et al., 1981) and a continuous line (C-10)

originating from fibroblasts transformed by SV40 was developed by Tan
(1981a). The superinduction procedure for production of interferon
from normal diploid fibroblasts has been adapted also to the MG-63
line. The fibroblastoid C-10 interferon was purified to homogeneity
by a combination of affinity chromatography on Concanavalin A and
adsorption chromatography on controlled-pore glass (Tan, 1981b).

PRODUCTION OF INTERFERON VIA RECOMBINANT DNA TECHNOLOGY

The evolution of molecular biology including the breakthroughs
summarized in the term "recombinant DNA technology" has been
intimately linked to the study of the bacterium E. coli and its
viruses. This prokaryotic organism has been a favorite for at least
three reasons. It has relatively simple genetics, a rapid growth
rate, and is well characterized generally. It was natural,
therefore, that E. coli should be the host into which the human
leukocyte interferon gene was inserted (Goeddel et al., 1979).

E. coli contains one large circular thread of chromosomal DNA
and several smaller circular units called plasmids. Plasmids
replicate independently of the chromosomal DNA and have become the
target of genetic engineering. With the help of special enzymes
called restriction endonucleases, the plasmid circles can be cut open
at specific sites allowing for selected DNA fragments to be spliced
into the opening. The covalent bonding between the ends of the
fragment and those of the open plasmid circle is accomplished by
another enzyme called DNA ligase. The DNA fragment to be inserted
may be derived from one of the three sources: (1) it may be
chemically synthesized to code for the known amino acid sequence of a
protein, (2) the DNA fragment may be excised from the chromosome of
interest, or (3) complementary DNA (cDNA) may be synthesized using
purified messenger RNA as a template and the enzyme reverse
transcriptase.

The new plasmid called the vector is introduced into the E. coli
host and the now transformed cells are grown on agar plates. The
selection of suitable colonies for growth in culture is known as the
cloning technique and allows for an essentially unlimited supply of
the donor DNA. Further engineering and reconstruction of the DNA
such as the addition of a promoter region provides for a high
expression of the new gene when the cells are grown in a shake flask
or a fermentor.

At the present time all recombinant interferons are being
produced in E. coli cells which have been described above. This
includes the subtypes of leukocyte interferon as well as fibroblast
interferon. E. coli has the limitation that its physiology does not
include an enzyme system for adding sugar side chains to proteins.
This is of no consequence in the production of the leukocyte

interferons which are not glycoproteins but it means that recombinant fibroblast interferon will be missing its natural carbohydrate moiety. The clinical significance of this simplification is not yet known. It may be possible to use a more complex eukaryotic host such as yeast (S. cerevisiae) which has the capability of glycosylating proteins. Yeast has already been used on a laboratory scale to express one of the leukocyte interferon clones (Goeddel et al., 1980) but the leukocyte interferons are generally not glycoproteins. Ongoing developments in molecular genetics can be expected to improve the yield for desired proteins whether in E. coli or other hosts. It has been reported for example that expression levels of recombinant proteins may reach as high as 30 to 50% of the soluble protein synthesized by the cell (Miozzari, 1981).

Large-scale fermentation technology has become increasingly more sophisticated since World War II when it became important for antibiotic production. Thus the way is open for kilogram quantities of recombinant micro-organisms to be produced. NIH guidelines for recombinant DNA research place some restrictions on scale up. Fermentations larger than ten liters are generally prohibited but may be carried out if physically contained. Harvesting of the cells must then be in ten liter aliquots unless the cells are killed. Cells once harvested by centrifugation are disrupted chemically or mechanically and the clarified extract passed through a series of steps including precipitation and chromatography (Fig. 1).

The goal of protein purification is to approach 100% homogeneity with the highest possible recovery. To achieve higher and higher purity, however, one must increase the number of purification steps and with each step there is an unavoidable loss of product. It is common experience that the price for higher purity is loss of yield. Newer adsorption media, however, based on high affinity as well as specificity between a covalently bound ligand and the protein in question have made it possible to achieve higher purity in a fewer steps. Enzyme inhibitors, substrate analogues, organic dyes, metal chelates, and even proteins have been successfully used as ligands in affinity purification of proteins. The most powerful affinity separation method, i.e. the one with the highest specificity for a single protein probably is immuno-affinity chromatography. A non-adsorbent polysaccharide bead such as agarose usually serves as a carrier on which purified antibodies, preferably monoclonal antibodies (Kwan et al., 1980) are immobilized. Monoclonal antibodies are monospecific and therefore highly selective for a single protein. It is thus conceptually possible to develop so-called single step purifications. Although the use of such a column is relatively simple, the preparation of the monoclonal antibodies is far from trivial. Four to six months may be required to establish a stable hybridoma which produces the antibodies. They then must be harvested, purified and chemically coupled to a support.

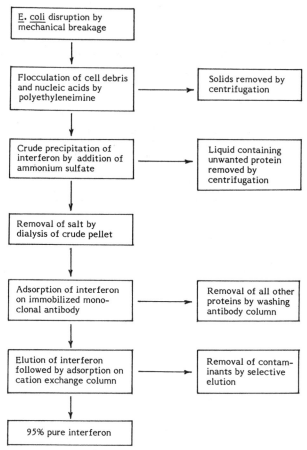

Fig. 1.   Immuno-affinity chromatography of recombinant leukocyte A
           interferon.

Chemically immobilized monoclonal antibodies have been used to
purify recombinant leukocyte A interferon (Staehelin, 1981). The
clear advantage of this method was high recovery (up to 81%) and high
specific activity (up to 3×10^8 units/mg, Table I). Since the
immobilized monoclonal antibody column can be washed and cycled a
number of times, the method is useful for preparing large quantities
of purified interferon.

Recombinant DNA technology provides an opportunity to make
hybrid interferons. Recombinants with common restriction
endonuclease sites can be cut and re-ligated with complementary
segments. By this means a series of active hybrids have been formed
on a laboratory scale (Streuli et al., 1981; Weck et al., 1981;
Rehberg et al., in press), but none is yet being produced for

TABLE I

Source, Specific Activity and Purity of Natural and
Recombinant Human Interferons Prepared on a Large Scale

Interferon Type	Source	Spec. Activity IU/mg	Purity %
IFN-alpha	leukocytes from normal blood	2.5×10^6 to 1.25×10^7	< 10
	lymphoblastoid (Namalva) cells	10^6 to 10^7	< 10
IFN-beta	diploid fibro- blasts (fore- skin, embryos)	2×10^7	20
rIFN-alpha A	transformed E. coli	3×10^8	> 95
rIFN-alpha D	same	5×10^7 to 1×10^8	> 95
rIFN-beta	same	1×10^8	> 98

clinical study. It may be possible through further genetic
engineering and reconstruction to tailor-make interferons with
desired activities but devoid of clinical side effects.

PRODUCT QUALITY CONTROL

     The production, testing, and marketing of human interferons,
whether derived from tissue culture or from transformed E. coli, is
subject to a variety of laws formulated in the Food, Drug, and
Cosmetic Act, the Public Health Safety Act, the Radiation Control for
Health and Safety Act, and the Fair Packaging and Labeling Act. The
detailed requirements for compliance with the various laws are
codified in the Code of Federal Regulations. The public regulatory
agency which exercises research and premarket approval authority is
the FDA. Safety, efficacy, purity, and identity of a product must be
demonstrated to the FDA before testing and marketing approval are
granted. Furthermore, all manufacturers must operate in conformance
with current Good Manufacturing Practices (GMP) that include properly

equipped facilities, adequately trained personnel, and appropriate
finished product examination, i.e. product quality control. GMP is
designed to protect the product from being compromised by
contamination during production. Final product examination assures
identity and purity as specified on the label.

Interferon identity whether natural or recombinant is first of
all established by an antiviral or cytopathic effect inhibition assay
as described by Armstrong (1981), Johnston et al. (1981), Familletti
et al. (1981b) and Rubinstein et al. (1981). Although this assay
defines interferon generally, a given preparation may be contaminated
with other biologically active components which will complicate final
product identity. Tissue culture cells, as described in a previous
section, are grown in complex media which contain many growth
supporting factors of animal and/or human origin. Contamination of
the final product, unless purified to highest levels, is unavoidable.
Natural human interferon preparations, hence, contain a large number
of biologically active factors, including lymphokines, colony
stimulating factor and many more of unknown activity. Clinical
trials with crude natural interferons, particularly at high doses,
are compromised by the presence of these factors which create side
effects masking the intrinsic activity of the interferons under
study. Patients administered interferons extracted from large pools
of donated blood run the risk of both common and slow virus infection
and, if derived from transformed cell lines, there is also the risk
of infection with oncogenic viruses. Crude natural interferon
preparations undoubtedly also contain impurities which originate from
the type of inducer used, e.g. Sendai virus and egg proteins (Sendai
virus is grown in chicken embryos), polyrIrC, and other ingredients
added during induction (Leong et al., 1979).

The establishment of product identity in the case of recombinant
interferons is somewhat easier because of the absence of the above
complex factors. Furthermore, the production process can be
monitored at the genomic as well as the final product level. For
example, the successful construction of the plasmid used for the
transformation of the E. coli can be verified by DNA sequencing.

In recent years analytical methods have been developed or
improved upon, which permit fast and accurate identification of the
finished purified product. The classic methods of N- and C-terminal
amino acid analysis in conjunction with proteolytic peptide mapping
have been greatly improved through recent developments in HPLC. The
resolving power of reverse phase HPLC columns permits analysis of
subnanomole quantities of complex peptide mixtures. In this way
information about the structure of the molecule can be gained in a
short time and with high reproducibility (Rubinstein et al., 1980).
Isoelectric focusing is yet another technique which provides
information about the identity as well as purity of the product. The
method is sensitive enough to discover single amino acid

substitutions if a change of the net charge is involved. The ultimate test for identity is amino acid sequencing. Sequencing of peptides and whole proteins is performed today on fully automated sequenators which allow penetration into the molecule from the N-terminus at a rate of three amino acids per day. The combined application of these methods in conjunction with radio- or enzyme immunoassays can unambiguously verify the structure of the final product.

We speak of 100% purity as an objective, knowing full well that no protein is ever absolutely pure. Any statement, therefore, about the level of purity should be accompanied by a description of the assay(s) used and its detection limit. In other words, purity is really defined by the assay(s). The type and number of assays employed will depend on knowledge of the production process and the substance classes which are likely to end up in the final product. It is customary to test for the absence of suspected contaminants as classes, e.g. micro-organisms, endotoxins (pyrogens), nucleic acids of viral or chromosomal origin, microbial proteins, etc.

Homogeneous is the term commonly used for highly purified protein which means only that other proteins are absent or negligible. Other contaminants mentioned above would not be detected in typical protein purity tests. The conventional method for the detection of proteinaceous impurities is electrophoresis in poly-acrylamide gel in presence of the denaturing detergent sodium dodecyl sulfate and the reducing agent mercaptoethanol. The method separates proteins on the basis of molecular weight differences. Protein bands are detected following electrophoresis by staining with Coomassie Blue which has a detection limit of 0.1 μg protein or about 1% of a μg load. Newer staining techniques with silver (Morrissey, 1981) have afforded sensitivities as much as 100 times greater than with Coomassie Blue (Oakley et al., 1980; Wray et al., 1981). Although the electrophoresis method is used for quantitative detection of impurities one has to keep in mind that it allows visualization of only protein impurities.

A newer alternative test of protein purity is size exclusion or reverse-phase HPLC which has high resolution and is much faster than electrophoresis. The HPLC identity test mentioned previously can also reveal information indirectly about protein purity. If impurities are present the terminal amino acid and sequence determination of fragments will be ambiguous.

CONCLUSION

Human interferon preparations available for clinical study vary widely (over a 100 fold range) in purity (Table I). The most purified preparations presently in clinical trial are those produced via recombinant DNA technology from transformed E. coli. For the first time dosage is no longer limited by the impurities present in crude concentrates of natural interferons and sufficient material is available to prove or disprove the usefulness of human interferons in the therapy of viral diseases and cancer.

The promise of recombinant DNA technology, however, far transcends the interferon field and on the horizon of current research and development we see the production of many other polypeptides of value in the therapy of human disease. It also can be anticipated that the new tool in the hands of the imaginative and gifted will be employed to uncover many of the riddles of life itself. Herein may lie its most rewarding application.

REFERENCES

Armstrong, J.A. 1981, Cytopathic effect inhibition assays for interferon: micro-culture plate assay, Methods in Enzymology, 78:381.

Berg, K., and Heron, I. 1981, Antibody affinity chromatography of human leukocyte interferon, Methods in Enzymology, 78:487.

Bodo, G. 1981, Procedures for large-scale production and partial purification of human interferon from lymphocyte (Namalva) cultures, Methods in Enzymology, 78:69.

Cantell, K., Hirvonen, S., Kauppinen, H.-L., and Myllyla, G. 1981a, Production of interferon in human leukocytes from normal donors with the use of Sendai virus, Methods in Enzymology, 78:29.

Cantell, K., Hirvonen, S., and Koistinen, V. 1981b, Partial purification of human leukocyte interferon on a large scale, Methods in Enzymology, 78:499.

de Ley, M., Van Damme, J., Claeys, H., Weening, H., Heine, J.W., Billiau, A., Vermylen, C., and de Somer, P. 1980, Interferon induced in human leukocytes by mitogens: production, partial purification and characterization, Eur. J. Immunol., 10:877.

Epstein, L.B. 1981, Induction and production of immune interferon by mitogen and antigen-stimulated purified lymphocytes cultured in the presence of macrophages, Methods in Enzymology, 78:147.

Familletti, P.C., Costello, L., Rose, C.A., and Pestka, S. 1981a, Induction, production, and concentration of interferon produced by a myeloblast culture, Methods in Enzymology, 78:83.

Familletti, P.C., Rubinstein, S., and Pestka, S. 1981b, A convenient and rapid cytopathic effect inhibition assay for interferon, Methods in Enzymology, 78:387.

Fleischmann, W.R., Jr., Georgiades, J.A., Osborne, L.C., and Johnson, H.M. 1979, Potentiation of interferon activity by mixed preparations of fibroblast and immune interferon, Infect. Immun., 26:248.

Friesen, H.-J., Stein, S., and Pestka, S. 1981, Purification of human fibroblast interferon by high-performance liquid chromatography, Methods in Enzymology, 78:430.

Giard, D.J., Loeb, D.H., Thilly, W.G., Wang, D.I.C., and Levine, D.W.
    1979, Human interferon production with diploid fibroblast cells
    grown on microcarriers, Biotechnol. Bioeng., 21:433.
Goeddel, D.V., Kleid, D.G., Bolivar, F., Heynecker, H.L., Yandura,
    D.G., Crea. R., Hirose, T., Kraszewski, A., Itakura, K., and
    Riggs, A.D. 1979, Expression in Escherichia coli of chemically
    synthesized genes for human insulin, Proc. Natl. Acad. Sci. USA,
    76:106.
Goeddel, D.V., Yelverton, E., Ullrich, A., Heyneker, H.L., Miozzari,
    G.F., Holmes, W., Seeburg, P.H., Dull, T., May, L., Stebbing,
    N., Crea, R., Maeda, S., McCandliss, R., Sloma, A., Tabor, J.M.,
    Gross, M., Familletti, P.C., and Pestka, S. 1980, Human
    leukocyte interferon produced by E. coli is biologically active,
    Nature, 287:411.
Gresser, I. 1961, Production of interferon by suspension of human
    leukocytes, Proc. Soc. Exp. Biol. Med., 108:799.
Havell, E.A., Yip, Y.K., and Vilcek, J. 1978, Characteristics of
    human lymphoblastoid (Namalva) interferon, J. Gen. Virol.,
    38:51.
Heine, K.J.W., and Billiau, A. 1981, Purification of human fibroblast
    interferon by adsorption on controlled-pore glass and
    zinc-chelate chromatography, Methods in Enzymology, 78:448.
Herschberg, R.D., Gusciora, E.G., Familletti, P.C., Rubinstein, S.,
    Rose, C.A., and Pestka, S. 1981, Induction and production of
    human interferon with human leukemic cells, Methods in
    Enzymology, 78:45.
Hobbs, D.S., Moschera, J., Levy, W.P., and Pestka, S. 1981,
    Purification of interferon produced in a culture of human
    granulocytes, Methods in Enzymology, 78:472.
Horowitz, B. 1981, Human interferon-properties, clinical application,
    and production, J. Parenteral Science and Technology, 35:223.
Johnson, H.M., Dianzani, F., and Georgiades, J.A. 1981, Large-scale
    induction and production of human and mouse immune interferon,
    Methods in Enzymology, 78:158.
Johnston, M.D., Finter, N.B., and Young, P.A. 1981, Dye uptake method
    for assay of interferon activity, Methods in Enzymology, 78:394.
Kenny, C., Moschera, J.A., and Stein, S. 1981, Purification of human
    fibroblast interferon produced in the absence of serum by
    Cibacron Blue F3GA-agarose and high-performance liquid
    chromatography, Methods in Enzymology, 78:435.
Klein, G., Dombos, L., and Gothoskar, B. 1972, Sensitivity of
    Epstein-Barr virus (EBV) producer and non-producer human lympho-
    blastoid cell lines to superinfection with EBV, Int. J. Cancer,
    10:44.
Klein, F., and Ricketts, R.T. 1981, Procedures for large-scale
    production and concentration of lymphoblastoid interferon,
    Methods in Enzymology, 78:75.
Knight, E. 1981, Purification of human fibroblast interferon prepared
    in the absence of serum, Methods in Enzymology, 78:417.
Koeffler, H.P., and Golde, D.W. 1978, Acute myelogenous leukemia: a
    human cell line responsive to colony-stimulating activity,
    Science, 200:1153.

Kwan, S.P., Yelton, D.E., and Scharff, M.D. 1980, Production of
    monoclonal antibodies, in: "Genetic Engineering: Principles and
    Methods", Vol. 2, J.K. Setlow and A. Hollander, eds., Plenum
    Press, New York.
Langford, M.P., Georgiades, J.A., Stanton, G.J., Danzoni, F., and
    Johnson, H.M. 1979, Large-scale production and physiochemical
    characterization of human immune interferon, Infect. Immun.,
    26:36.
Lin, L.S., and Stewart, W.E., II. 1981, Purification of human
    leukocyte interferon by two-dimensional polyacrylamide gel
    electrophoresis, Methods in Enzymology, 78:481.
Leong, S.S., Horoszewicz, J.S., and Carter, W.A. 1979, Human
    fibroblast interferon (HFIF): antiproliferative activity of
    crude and purified preparations, Abstr. Amer. Soc. Microbiol.,
    p.277.
Leong, S.S., and Horoszewicz, J.S. 1981, Production and preparations
    of human fibroblast interferon for clinical trials,,Methods in
    Enzymology, 78:87.
Miozzari, G.F. 1981, Strategies for obtaining expression of peptide
    hormones in E. coli in: "Insulins, Growth Hormone, and
    Recombinant DNA Technology", J.L. Gueriguian, ed., Raven Press,
    New York.
Mizrahi, A. 1981, Production of human lymphoblastoid (Namalva)
    interferon, Methods in Enzymology, 78:54.
Morrissey, J.H. 1981, Silver stain for proteins in polyacrylamide
    gels: a modified procedure with enhanced uniform sensitivity,
    Anal. Biochem., 117:307.
Oakley, B.R., Kirsch, D.R., and Morris, N.R. 1980, A simplified
    ultrasensitive silver stain for detecting proteins in
    polyacrylamide gels, Anal. Biochem., 105:361.
Pritchett, R., Pedersen, M., and Keiff, E. 1976, Complexity of EBV
    homologous DNA in continuous lymphoblastoid cell lines,
    Virology, 74:227..
O'Malley, J.A. 1981, Affinity chromatography of human immune
    interferon, Methods in Enzymology, 78:540.
Rehberg, E., Kelder, B., Hoal, E.G., and Pestka, S. Specific
    molecular activities of recombinant and hybrid leukocyte
    interferons, J. Biol. Chem. (in press).
Rubinstein, M., Stein, S., and Udenfriend, S. 1980, Fluorometric
    methods for analysis of proteins and peptides: principles and
    applications, Hormonal Proteins and Peptides, 9:1.
Rubinstein, S., Familletti, P.C., and Pestka, S. 1981, Convenient
    assay for interferons, J. Virol., 37:755.
Rubinstein, M., and Pestka, S. 1981, Purification and
    characterization of human leukocyte interferons by high-
    performance liquid chromatography, Methods in Enzymology,
    78:464.
Staehelin, T., Hobbs, D.S., Kung, H.-F., Lai, C.-Y, and Pestka, S.
    1981, Purification and characterization of recombinant human
    leukocyte interferon (rIFN-alpha D) with monoclonal antibodies,
    J. Biol. Chem., 256:9750.

Strander, H., and Cantell, K. 1966, Production of interferon by human leukocytes in vitro, Ann. Med. Exp. Biol. Fenn., 44:265.

Strander, H., Morgensen, K.E., and Cantell, K. 1975, Production of human lymphoblastoid interferon, J. Clin. Microbiol., 116.

Streuli, M., Hall, A., Boll, W., Stewart, W.E., II, Nagata, S., and Weissmann, C. 1981, Target cell specificity of two species of human interferons-alpha produced in Escherichia coli and of hybrid molecules derived from them, Proc. Natl. Acad. Sci. USA, 78:2848.

Tan, Y.H. 1981a, Induction and production of human interferon with a continuous line of modified fibroblast, Methods in Enzymology, 78:422.

Tan, Y.H. 1981b, Purification of human fibroblast interferon prepared from modified fibroblasts, Methods in Enzymology, 78:422.

Van Damme, J., and Billiau, A. 1981, Large-scale production of human fibroblast interferon, Methods in Enzymology, 78:101.

Von Wussow, P., Chen, Y.-S., Wiranowska-Stewart, M., and Stewart, W.E., II, 1982, Induction of human gamma interferon in lymphoid cells by Staphylococcus enterotoxin B: partial purification, J. Interferon Res., 2:11.

Waldman, A.A., Miller, R.S., Familletti, P.C., Rubinstein, S., and Pestka, S. 1981, Induction and production of interferon with human leukocytes from normal donors with the use of Newcastle disease virus, Methods in Enzymology, 78:39.

Weck, P.K., Apperson, S., Stebbing, N., Gray, P.W., Leung, D., Shepard, H.M., and Goeddel, D.V. 1981, Antiviral activities of hybrids of two major human leukocyte interferons, Nucleic Acid Res., 9:6153.

Wray, W., Boulikas, T., Wray, V.P., and Hancock, R. 1981, Silver staining of proteins in polyacrylamide gels, Anal. Biochem., 118:197.

Yip, Y.K., Pang, R.H.L., Urban, C., and Vilcek, J. 1981, Partial purification and characterization of human gamma (immune) interferon, Proc. Natl. Acad. Sci. USA, 78:1601.

Zoon, K.C. 1981, Purification and characterization of human interferon from lymphoblastoid (Namalva) cultures, Methods in Enzymology, 78:457.

BIOCHEMICAL ACTIONS

BRYAN R.G. WILLIAMS

Division of Infectious Diseases, Department of
Paediatrics, The Hospital for Sick Children, Toronto
Ontario, Canada

Recent studies have shown that the human, mouse and bovine
interferon (IFN) families consist of various gene products which may
be both functionally and structurally heterogeneous. For example,
the existence of multiple gene products of the IFN α family suggests
that there may be specific roles for different molecular subtypes
during stages of differentiation and development (Nagata et al.,
1980). The capacity of interferon to exhibit such diverse activities
is reflected by the multiplicity of biochemical responses detected in
interferon-treated cells (Gordon and Minks, 1981; Borden and Ball,
1982; Lengyel, 1982). Most interferons share the same biochemical
activities but quantitative differences are apparent among molecular
subtypes as reflected by the differential activity on cells from
different species. Although classically described as antiviral
agents, the biochemical changes interferons elicit in cells are not
selectively antiviral but sufficiently diverse to affect both viral
and cellular metabolism. Nevertheless, the recent major advances in
understanding the mechanism of action of interferon have come mainly
from studies on the inhibition of viral replication.

Cells exposed to interferon can develop an antiviral state in
which the growth of many RNA and DNA viruses is inhibited. This
state depends on RNA and protein synthesis and is a transient
phenomenon. Depending on cell type and virus, the inhibition may be
directed at viral RNA synthesis or methylation, viral protein
synthesis, uncoating of the virus or virus maturation and release.
While a single mechanism may result in inhibition of virus growth it
is likely that multiple sites of action are involved and that
different mechanisms are utilized. The importance of specific
mechanisms may be dictated by the nature of the replicative cycle of
the virus. These antiviral mechanisms may also contribute to the

33

cell growth inhibitory and immunoregulatory activities of interferons.

EARLY BIOCHEMICAL EVENTS INITIATED BY INTERFERON TREATMENT

All the biochemical activities of interferon (Table I) are initiated by specific binding to the surface receptor on the cell (Aguet, 1980). Competitive binding studies have indicated that α and β interferons share the same receptor(s) which is different from the γ receptor (Branca and Baglioni, 1981). After binding, human interferon is internalized and degraded by cells, a process that may involve the cytoskeleton (Branca and Baglioni, 1982). However, this internalization may not be necessary for activity as mouse interferon is released intact from the cells.

The earliest biochemical change effected by interferon is a marked increase in the intracellular concentration of cyclic GMP which occurs within minutes of exposure to interferon and can be inhibited by aspirin or by calcium limitation (Rochette-Egly and Tovey, 1982). The inhibition of cyclic GMP increase does not affect

TABLE I

Changes in Cellular Biochemical Functions
Following Interferon Treatment

Gene Expression

2-5A synthetase	2'-phosphodiesterase
endonuclease	HLA-ABC
protein kinase	β_2 microglobulin

Augmentation of Activity

arylhydrocarbon hydroxylase	type IV collagenase
prostaglandin E_2, F_2	cyclic AMP
histamine	cyclic GMP
tRNA methylase	

Depression of Activity

glycosyltransferase	hexose monophosphate shunt
glucocorticoid inducible enzymes	membrane unsaturated fatty
ornithine decarboxylase	acid content
s-adenosyl methionine decarboxylase	thymidine transport
hepatic cytochrome P-450-linked	protein phosphatases
monooxygenases	

the establishment of the antiviral state. However, the elevation of cyclic AMP levels, which occurs some hours after interferon treatment, may contribute to the growth inhibitory effects of interferon. Recent analysis of cyclic AMP responsive and un-responsive transformed macrophages has indicated that interferon-mediated stimulation of phagocytosis and inhibition of growth occurs through increased intracellular levels of cyclic AMP. The antiviral activity of interferon in these cells was found to be independent of cyclic AMP (Schneck et al., 1982). These results support an earlier study which correlated growth inhibition with increase in intracellular cyclic AMP levels in very different human cell lines (Fuse and Kuwata, 1978). The mechanisms underlying the changes in cyclic nucleotide levels are not known. The establishment of the antiviral state and the anticellular activities of interferon results in the synthesis of several new messenger RNAs and proteins. Although this is concomitant with several other cellular biochemical changes (Table I), few have been identified with any functional activity. It is probable that many of the enzymatic changes detected in cells treated with interferon are secondary effects. Never-theless, some may be particularly important for very different reasons. For example, the interferon-mediated depression of hepatic cytochrome P-450-linked monooxygenases (which can be demonstrated with highly purified recombinant interferons in addition to interferon inducers) can result in elevated serum drug levels in combined interferon-acyclovir therapy (Mannering et al., 1980; Singh et al., 1982).

Recently, another study has demonstrated that interferon can significantly elevate levels of type IV collagenase production by human sarcoma cells (Siegal et al., 1982). This has been correlated with an enhancement of the invasiveness of these cells for human basement membrane independent of any effect on cell growth. There is as yet no evidence that this phenomenon extends to the cells or tumors in vivo; however, this study has important implications for the clinical use of interferon.

Induced enzyme activity can either be augmented, as in the case of arylhydrocarbon hydroxylase, or depressed, as in glucocorticoid-induced glutamine synthetase, glycerol-3-phosphate dehydrogenase and tyrosine amino transferase (Nebert and Friedman, 1973; Beck et al., 1974; Illinger et al., 1976; Matsuno et al., 1976). The inhibition of ornithine decarboxylase (ODC) activity by interferon may be related to the induction of a polyamine-dependent protein kinase activity but the contribution of ODC inhibition of interferon action remains obscure (Sreevalsen et al., 1980; Sekar et al., 1982). Similarly, the effect of increased prostaglandin synthesis after interferon treatment and the significance of results showing that cyclooxygenase inhibition blocks development of the antiviral state are not clear (Yaron et al., 1977; Fitzpatrick and Stringfellow, 1980).

Of the mRNAs induced in interferon treated cells, only that for
2-5A synthetase had been identified until recently. It has now been
demonstrated that there are large increases in HLA-A, B, C and β_2
microglobulin mRNAs following interferon treatment (Fellous et al.,
1982). These would account for the increase in HLA, A, B, C and β_2
microglobulin antigen expression in cells exposed to interferon. The
expression of Fcγ receptors on T cells is also increased by
interferon. This enhanced expression of cell surface antigens may be
an important factor contributing to the immunoregulatory effects of
interferon. Interestingly, the increase in HLA mRNA synthesis occurs
within one hr of interferon treatment and precedes the increases in
2-5A synthetase mRNA.

Interferon can inhibit the incorporation of exogenous thymidine
into DNA. While this may reflect a lower rate of DNA synthesis it is
now apparent that the rates of a number of deoxynucleoside metabolic
steps may be affected. For example, both transport of thymidine and
phosphorylation can be inhibited in interferon-treated cells (Gewart
et al., 1981). The alteration in membrane transport is one of many
cell surface changes resulting from interferon treatment. The
contribution of these changes to the biological effects of interferon
are probably important but the biochemistry underlying the changes is
yet to be elucidated. However, there is now considerable evidence
that the novel enzyme activities induced in interferon-treated cells
(Table I) play an important role in mediating the antiviral activity
of interferon.

INTERFERON-INDUCED ENZYME ACTIVITIES INVOLVED IN PROTEIN SYNTHESIS
INHIBITION

A comparison of the translational and transcriptional activity
of cell-free extracts from untreated and interferon-treated cells has
identified several changes induced by interferon treatment. These
include effects on mRNA methylation (Sen et al., 1977), inactivation
of some tRNA species (Sen et al., 1976), inhibition of glycosylation
(Maheshwari et al., 1980) and enhanced sensitivity to protein
synthesis inhibition by double-stranded RNA (dsRNA) (Kerr et al.,
1974). The marked inhibitory effects of dsRNA on protein synthesis
in extracts from interferon-treated cells correlates with the
sensitivity of interferon-treated cells to the cytotoxic effects of
dsRNA (Stewart et al., 1972). Detailed studies of this phenomenon
have led to major advances in understanding the biochemistry of
interferon action. Two major dsRNA-dependent enzyme activities are
involved: an oligo- nucleotide synthetase, which makes a series of
2'-5'-linked oligonucleotides from adenosine triphosphate and a
protein kinase. These enzyme activities are sufficient to mediate
the inhibition of protein synthesis by dsRNA in extracts from
interferon-treated cells. Therefore, they probably play an important
role in the antiviral activity of interferon and may also be involved
in some of the regulatory functions of interferon.

THE dsRNA-DEPENDENT PROTEIN KINASE

The incubation of extracts from interferon-treated cells with μg P-32 ATP and dsRNA results in the phosphorylation of at least two proteins. One termed P1 has a molecular weight of 67,000 to 72,000 daltons depending on cell type. The other is a 38,000 dalton peptide identified as the α subunit of the protein synthesis initiation factor eIF-2 (Lebleu et al., 1976; Roberts et al., 1976) (Fig. 1).

The protein kinase activity has been partially purified from interferon-treated cells and purification studies suggest that the phosphorylation of P1 protein probably represents an auto-phosphorylation (Sen et al., 1978; Zilberstein et al., 1978). There is no dependence on cAMP. In addition to the α subunit of eIF-2, some histone species can also act as a substrate for phosphorylation (Roberts et al., 1976). Recently Sekar et al. (1982) described a protein kinase activity in interferon-treated cells that is stimulated by polyamines. This activity co-purifies with the dsRNA-dependent kinase and the two probably represent a single enzyme activity.

Studies on interferon induced protein kinase activities can be complicated by protein phosphatase activity present in cell extracts which can dephosphorylate the P1 protein and eIF-2 subunit (Zilberstein et al., 1978). 1979). This phosphatase activity can be inhibited by dsRNA (Epstein et al., 1980). Some studies have found that the purified kinase activity may not be dependent on dsRNA (Sen et al., 1978). This suggests that the purification scheme may have eliminated dsRNA-binding phosphatase activity. The role of phosphatase appears complex, as was emphasized by a recent study showing a dramatic reduction in the level of general protein

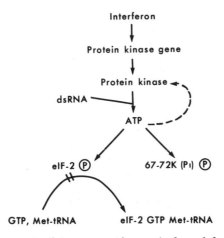

Fig. 1. The protein kinase pathway induced by interferon.

phosphorylation in the human lymphoblastoid Daudi cell line in
response to interferon treatment.

A dsRNA-dependent protein kinase which phosphorylates eIF-2 has
also been purified from rabbit reticulocyte lysates (Farrell et al.,
1977; Levin et al., 1980). Both this enzyme and the interferon-
induced kinase phosphorylate the smallest subunit of eIF-2 at sites
that are indistinguishable from those phosphorylated by the
reticulocyte hemin-regulated kinase (Samuel, 1979). The net result
of these kinase activities is the inhibition of peptide chain
initiation by preventing binding of methionyl tRNA to native 40's
ribosomal subunits (Farrell et al., 1977; Lewis et al., 1978). This
can be overcome by the addition of purified eIF-2 to inhibited cell-
free protein synthesizing systems. Phosphorylation of the α subunit
of eIF-2 appears to prevent the interaction between eIF-2 and an
eIF-2 stimulating protein (SP) which is essential for the maximal
ternary complex formation (eIF-2-GTP-Met-tRNA) which binds to the 40s
ribosome (Clemens et al., 1982; Siekierka et al., 1982) (Fig. 1).

The role of protein kinase in mediating interferon activity is
not clear. Phosphorylation of histones may contribute to the
alterations in gene expression and DNA synthesis seen in interferon-
treated cells but this remains to be demonstrated. That the kinase
activity is not just an in vitro artefact is shown by the finding
that dsRNA added to intact IFN-treated cells results in Pl protein
phosphorylation (Gupta, 1979). Furthermore, a protein kinase
activity which can phosphorylate Pl and added eIF-2 has been detected
in interferon-treated EMC virus infected cells (Golgher et al.,
1980). This activity is not dependent on dsRNA and indicates prior
activation of the kinase by dsRNA in viral replication complex. The
relative importance of protein kinase activity in mediating the antiviral activity of interferon is not yet confirmed. There is some
evidence that the reticulocyte kinase is activated at lower dsRNA
concentrations than 2-5A synthetase but that phosphorylation is
reversed at high dsRNA concentrations (Williams et al., 1979).
Therefore, the kinase may be active early in virus infection or
important when dsRNA is only a minor component of viral replication
complexes.

THE 2-5A SYNTHETASE SYSTEM

The incubation of interferon-treated cell extracts with ATP and
dsRNA activates the 2',5'-oligoadenylate synthetase (2-5A synthetase)
in addition to the protein kinase (Roberts et al., 1976). This
enzyme can be bound to dsRNA-agarose affinity columns and used to
synthesize the novel series of oligonucleotides with a general
structure of ppp(A2'p)nA where n=2 to ≤4 (Hovanessian et al., 1977;
Ball and White, 1978; Kerr and Brown, 1978). These are collectively
referred to as 2-5A. The 2'-5'-phosphodiester bonds are unique for

biologically synthesized material. While the dimer, trimer and tetramer are the most abundant forms, higher oligomers can be produced particularly if highly active, concentrated enzyme preparations are used (Martin et al., 1979; Justesen et al., 1980b; Minks et al., 1980; Samanta et al., 1980). The trimer, tetramer and pentamer have similar biological activities although the trimer is inactive in reticulocyte lysates (Williams et al., 1979). The dimer and non-phosphorylated "core" ((A2'p)nA) are inactive as protein synthesis inhibitors in all in vitro systems tested (Martin et al., 1979; Williams et al., 1979).

Other nucleotide triphosphates can act as nucleotidyl donors when mixed with ATP, dsRNA and 2-5A synthetase preparations or when added to preformed 2-5A oligomers (Ball, 1980; Justesen et al., 1980a). Cordycepin 5'-triphosphate (3'-deoxyadenosine) is also a substrate for the synthetase (Doetsch et al., 1981). Furthermore, in vitro, the synthetase can 2' adenylate important metabolites such as NAD+, ADP ribose and A5'p4S'A (Ball and White, 1979).

There is a widespread distribution of 2-5A synthetase in a variety of cells and tissues from mammals and birds. Although uninduced levels vary widely, treatment with interferon results in increase of ten to 10,000-fold (Stark et al., 1979). These increases can occur as early as three hours after exposure to interferons reaching a maximum around 24 hr (Ball, 1979; Kimchi et al., 1979). The inhibition of this response by actinomycin D and cycloheximide and detection of increased amounts of mRNA for the synthetase indicate that the induction of synthetase gene expression occurs after interferon treatment (Shulman and Revel, 1980). The induction of synthetase activity is transient and enzyme levels decline when interferon is removed. This decrease appears to require active protein synthesis as synthetase activity can be stabilized by cycloheximide treatment (Gupta et al., 1981). Interestingly, virus infection after interferon treatment can result in a further stimulation of enzyme synthesis (L.A. Ball, personal communication). Changes in growth conditions and the aging of cells in vitro can enhance the inducibility of the synthetase by interferon (Stark et al., 1979). Glucocorticoids alone may also induce enzyme activity (Krishnan and Baglioni, 1980a).

The 2-5A synthetase has been purified to apparent homogeneity by using either interferon-treated mouse Ehrlich ascites tumor cells or Hela cells as the enzyme source (Dougherty et al., 1980). The apparent molecular weight is 100,000 to 105,000 daltons. However, the enzyme from chick cells appears to be about 56,000 daltons (Ball, 1980). The translation of human lymphoblastoid cell (Namalva) mRNA for 2-5A synthetase in reticulocyte lysates suggests a much smaller enzyme than is present in Hela cells (Ball, 1980). The molecular cloning of the synthetase gene should resolve these discrepancies (Lengyel et al., 1982).

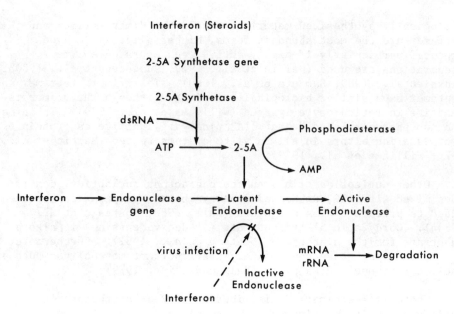

Fig. 2.   The 2-5A synthetase pathway induced by interferon.

The purified enzyme has an absolute requirement for dsRNA and this cannot be substituted by dsDNA or RNA-DNA hybrids (Ball and White, 1978; Minks et al., 1979). However, regions of secondary structure in some single stranded RNA molecules may be sufficient to activate the enzyme and viral replication intermediates containing both single and double-stranded RNA are good activators (Nilsen and Baglioni, 1979). The double stranded regions present in hetero-geneous nuclear RNA can also activate the synthetase (Nilsen et al., 1982).

The oligomers of 2-5A inhibit protein synthesis by activating a latent endoribonuclease (Baglioni et al., 1978; Clemens and Williams, 1978) (Fig. 2). This activation is transient as 2-5A is rapidly degraded by a 2'-phosphodiesterase to ATP and AMP (Williams et al., 1978). The basal level of phosphodiesterase is usually relatively high but may increase after the treatment of some cells with interferon and can vary significantly among cell lines (Kimchi et al., 1979; Silverman et al., 1982). For example, Hela cells have a higher level than rabbit reticulocytes or mouse Ehrlich ascites tumor cells (Silverman et al., 1981).

The activation of the endonuclease requires binding of 2-5A to the enzyme (Slattery et al., 1979). The radioactive analogue $ppp(A^{2'}p)3A(^{32}p)pCp$ also binds and this has been utilized in developing competition assays for 2-5A and for affinity labelling of a polypeptide of about 85,000 daltons (Knight et al., 1980; Wreschner

et al., 1982). This is presumed to be the endonuclease but remains
to be firmly established. Once activated, the nuclease in both crude
and partially purified preparations cleaves RNA on the 3'-side of UA
or UU sequences yielding UpAp- or UpUp-terminated products (Wreschner
et al., 1981). The activated nuclease also cleaves ribosomal RNA
present in intact ribosomes to yield discrete products. Recent
experiments have shown that in some cells the endonuclease levels may
be increased by up to ten-fold by interferon treatment thus
indicating a further level of control for the 2-5A system (Fig. 2).

ROLE OF THE 2-5A SYSTEM IN MEDIATING THE ANTIVIRAL ACTIVITY OF
INTERFERON

The 2-5A system has been demonstrated to function in vivo and
several criteria suggest that it is a major contributor to the
antiviral activity of interferon. Interferon-treated cells
synthesize 2-5A in response to virus infection and discrete ribosomal
RNA cleavages characteristic of 2-5A-activated endonuclease activity
can be demonstrated (Williams et al., 1979; Wreschner et al., 1981).
Increased levels of 2-5A and polysome degradation can also be seen in
interferon-treated cells exposed to dsRNA (Nilsen et al., 1981).
Cells deficient in latent endonuclease activity when treated with
interferon replicate EMC and VSV viruses normally despite enhanced
2-5A synthetase levels (Epstein et al., 1981; Panet et al., 1981).
When deliberately introduced into suitably treated cells, 2-5A
inhibits protein synthesis (Williams and Kerr, 1978; Hovanessian et
al., 1979). This inhibition also involves activation of an
endonuclease and is transient when low concentrations of 2-5A are
employed (Williams et al., 1979). Virus replication can be inhibited
when 2-5A is introduced into virus-infected cells. In contrast,
cells lacking the activatable endonuclease activity, introduced to
2-5A fail to inhibit protein synthesis and do not protect from virus
infection (Panet et al., 1981). Since normal levels of protein
kinase can be induced by interferon treating these cells P1 and eIF-2
phosphorylation are not sufficient for antiviral activity. Clearly
in some virus-cell combinations the 2-5A system plays an important
role in mediating the antiviral activity of interferons.

The 2-5A activated endonuclease show no specificity for viral
mRNA. Host messenger and ribosomal RNA cleavages are catalyzed by
the endonuclease both in vitro and in vivo. Furthermore, basal
levels of the 2-5A synthetase vary widely in different cells and
under different culture conditions with little apparent effect on
viral replication. Nevertheless, some selectivity can be argued for
the 2-5A system. For example, if total cellular metabolism is
inhibited in interferon-treated virus-infected cells the cell may die
but produce few viral progeny. This would effectively limit the
infection. Alternatively, the transient nature of the 2-5A system
may efficiently destroy the virus but allow the cell to recover

ultimately. It is also possible that localized activation of the
2-5A system might occur around replicating viral intermediates
containing dsRNA regions. Certainly in vitro, it can be demonstrated
that single-stranded RNAs covalently joined to dsRNA segments are
degraded preferentially over identical RNA not bound to dsRNA by
virtue of 2-5A system activation (Nilsen and Baglioni, 1979).
Clearly, the complexing of the synthetase and endonuclease and the
proximity of the 2'-phosphodiesterase could effectively
compartmentalize the 2-5A system in vivo.

Recently, a number of anomalies have arisen from studies of the
2-5A system in different cell lines. Some cells respond to
interferon by inducing the 2-5A synthetase but not the kinase. In
other cells the reverse is the case. This was first noted in mouse
embryonal carcinoma cells where interferon failed to induce the
protein kinase and did not inhibit VSV replication (Wood and
Hovanessian, 1979). However, resistance to EMC infection developed
along with 2-5A synthetase induction (Nilsen et al., 1980). In mouse
fibroblasts the opposite occurred; protein kinase and resistance to
VSV infection were induced by interferon but 2-5A synthetase activity
remained at basal levels (Hovanessian et al., 1981). In contrast to
these results, in some strains of human fibroblasts, resistance to
VSV can be demonstrated by interferon in the absence of protein
kinase induction but where 2-5A synthetase is induced normally
(Holmes and Gupta, 1982). Therefore, resistance to VSV infection can
be mediated by the 2-5A system or the protein kinase. In a strain of
human fibroblasts where neither 2-5A synthetase nor protein kinase
levels are affected by interferon resistance to VSV replication
probably occurs by inhibition of viral protein glycosylation (Meurs
et al., 1981). A similar conclusion can be drawn from studies where
gangliosides inhibited interferon induction of 2-5A synthetase but
did not prevent the development of resistance tp VSV infection
(Krishmamurti et al., 1982).

Recently, a further level of control has been added to the 2-5A
synthetase system. In EMC virus-infected cells the 2-5A activated
endonuclease has been found to be inhibited or inactivated. This
effect can be prevented by pretreating cells with interferon (Cayley
et al., 1982) (Fig. 2). These results explain the normal levels of
virus replication seen in cells with high basal levels of 2-5A
synthetase. They also suggest that prevention of virus-mediated
inhibition of the 2-5A-activated endonuclease by pretreatment with
interferon may be important than the absolute levels of 2-5A
synthetase. The mechanism of EMC virus-mediated inhibition of the
2-5A-activated endonuclease has not yet been determined.

A WIDER REGULATORY FUNCTION FOR THE 2-5A SYSTEM

The 2-5A synthetase has been found in a wide variety of
mammalian and avian cells and tissues at different levels which

usually increase in response to interferon treatment. There is even
a recent report of a 2-5A synthetase-like activity in plants
(Orchansky et al., 1982).

The common occurrence of 2-5A synthetase, its ability to utilize
important metabolites as substrates and the potential for the
complete 2-5A system to be compartmentalized and closely regulated
have led to increased interest in a possible wider role. This could
be either in mediating the growth inhibitory or immunomodulatory
effects of intereferon or in regulating cellular activities which are
distinct from interferon action. Despite intensive efforts no
alternative product of the synthetase has been detected _in vivo_. The
only products identified to date as occurring naturally are
ppp(A2'p)nA and (A2'p)nA (Williams et al., 1980). Interestingly, the
latter (the non-phosphorylated core of 2-5A), which is inactive as an
inhibitor of protein synthesis _in vitro_, can inhibit DNA synthesis
and cell growth (Martin et al., 1981). Both 2-5A and core have been
detected in interferon-treated cells although levels are low in the
absence of virus infection (Williams et al., 1980). This suggests
that the synthetase can be activated by a naturally occurring
component which provides the appropriate dsRNA structural
requirements and furthermore, that the 2-5A system is operative in
other than an antiviral state. Furthermore evidence for alternative
functions comes from the demonstration that the antimitogenic
activity of interferon against concanavalin A-stimulated
blastogenesis can be mimicked by 2-5A core (Kimchi et al., 1981).
This antimitogenic effect of core appears to be mediated by an
inhibition of the mitogen-dependent increase in protein synthesis
preferentially affecting histones (Kimchi et al., 1981). The
inhibition may involve RNase activation after core becomes rephos-
phorylated (a 5' tri- or diphosphate is essential for this) or
alternatively, the core may competitively inhibit the 2'-phospho-
diesterase resulting in an increased level of intracellular 2-5A.
Certainly, the ratio of 2'-phosphodiesterase to 2-5A synthetase can
vary in cells culture under various growth conditions but
measurements demonstrating changes in endogenous 2-5A levels under
these conditions have not been reported (Kimchi et al., 1981).

The possible involvement of 2-5A in the growth-inhibitory
effects of interferon on the very sensitive Daudi line of human
lymphoblastoid cells has been investigated using sensitive
radio-binding and radioimmunoassays for 2-5A (Silverman et al.,
1982). No 2-5A or alternative products in the concentration range
limit of the assays could be detected. There was also no evidence
for 2-5A mediated ribosomal RNA cleavage in interferon treated cells.
However, there was a two-fold increase in 2-5A-dependent RNase in
interferon treated wild type Daudi cells when compared to a line
selected for its resistance to the growth inhibitory effects of
interferon. Therefore, it is possible that the production of low
levels of 2-5A coupled with localized activation of elevated RNase is

affecting cells metabolism. In support of this, a line of NIH3T3 cells chronically infected with murine leukemia virus and resistant to the growth inhibitory effects of interferon, is deficient in 2-5A-dependent RNase activity (Panet et al., 1981). Overall, however, it has yet to be conclusively demonstrated that the 2-5A system plays any role in the growth-inhibitory effects of interferon or is involved in controlling cell growth or differentiation.

CLINICAL SIGNIFICANCE OF INTERFERON INDUCED ENZYME ACTIVITIES

As easily identifiable interferon-induced gene products the 2-5A synthetase and protein kinase provide useful markers for the presence of interferon activity in vivo. Furthermore, the detection of elevated levels of these enzyme activities during virus infection provides direct evidence for the triggering of the interferon system as a means of host defence. This has now been demonstrated in both the animal model and human infections. One of the early studies showed that both 2-5A synthetase activity and interferon appeared in the trigeminal ganglia of mice during the acute phase of HSV infection after cheek skin inoculation (Sokawa et al., 1980). Interferon diminished more rapidly than the synthetase which declined with the disappearance of the virus. The activities of both interferon and synthetase were undetectable after the conversion from the acute to the latent phase of infection. These results suggest that interferon acts through the 2-5A system to suppress virus multiplication during the acute productive phase of HSV infection.

The level of 2-5A synthetase is enhanced in the spleens and sera from mice infected with EMC virus (Krishnan and Baglioni, 1980b). The enzyme level also increases in livers and spleens from mice injected with Newcastle Disease Virus polyrI·rC or interferon. Phosphorylation of P1 and the presence of histone kinase activity were reported in this study. Administration of anti-interferon globulin before dsRNA injection blocked the induction of both synthetase and kinase activities. In newborn mice infected at birth with lymphocytic choriomeningitis virus (LCMV) there were large increases in 2-5A synthetase levels (Hovanessian and Riviere, 1980). The pathogenesis of LCMV infection in newborn mice has been linked to interferon production and it is possible that the liver cell degeneration seen may involve the activity of the 2-5A system.

In man interferon can be detected in serum and tissue during acute viral infection. However, the levels are often low and transient, and there is often a poor correlation between interferon and virus infection. On the other hand, the levels of 2-5A synthetase are elevated in extracts of peripheral blood mononuclear cells (PBM) from virus-infected patients (Schattner et al., 1981; Williams and Read, 1981). Moreover, these levels remain elevated throughout the course of disease and often reflect the site and severity of infection (Williams et al., 1982). In some infections the assay facilitates diagnosis and can be used to indicate a viral involvement in diseases of unknown etiology. It is interesting that the basal levels of 2-5A synthetase in PBM from normal healthy subjects is relatively high. Whether this reflects continuing exposure to interferon-inducing agents or indicates a role for interferon in lymphocyte differentiation remains to be determined (Kimchi, 1981).

Human plasma samples exhibit a protein kinase activity which appears to be identical to the P1 kinase (Hovanessian et al., 1982). The levels vary among individuals but remain constant in an individual. Patients treated with the adjuvant poly A·poly U as part of therapy for breast cancer show an enhanced level of kinase activity. There was no detectable interferon activity in these plasmas although studies in mice suggest that interferon is responsible for enhanced P1 kinase activity. The assay of plasma P1 kinase provides another simple test for the activation of the interferon system in vivo.

Recently, the synthetase assay has been demonstrated to be useful in determining patient response to interferon therapy (Schattner et al., 1981; Merritt et al., 1982). Changes in enzyme levels can be correlated with interferon administration. It is not known whether there is a direct relationship between enzyme induction in PBM and response to interferon therapy. However, this enzyme assay presents an opportunity to correlate the response of PBM to interferon treatment in vitro before therapy with changes in enzyme levels occurring during interferon administration. Eventually, it may be possible to use the assay as part of a screening process to preselect patients who will respond to interferon therapy.

ACKNOWLEDGEMENTS

B.R.G. Williams is an MRC (Canada) Scholar and his research activities are supported by grants from the Canadian MRC and NCI.

DEDICATION

This chapter is dedicated to the memory of Vivien Williams, 1949-1982.

REFERENCES

Aguet, M. 1980, High-affinity binding of ^{125}I-labelled mouse
     interferon to a specific cell surface receptor, Nature, 284:459.
Baglioni, C., Minks, M.A., and Maroney, P.A. 1978, Interferon action
     may be mediated by activation of a nuclease by pppA2'p5'A2'p5'A,
     Nature, 273:684.

Ball, L.A. 1979, Induction of 2'5'-oligoadenylate synthetase activity and a new protein by chick interferon, Virology, 94:282.

Ball, L.A. 1980, Induction, purification, and properties of 2'5' oligoadenylate synthetase, Ann. N.Y. Acad. Sci., 350:486.

Ball, L.A., and White, C.N. 1978, Oligonucleotide inhibitor of protein synthesis made in extracts of interferon-treated chick embryo cells: comparison with the mouse low molecular weight inhibitor, Proc. Natl. Acad. Sci. USA, 75:1167.

Ball, L.A., and White, C.N. 1979, Induction, purification, and properties of 2'5'-oligoadenylate synthetase, in: "Regulation of Macromolecular Synthesis", G. Koch and D. Richter, eds., Academic Press, New York, pp. 303-317.

Beck, G., Poindron, P., Illinger, D., Beck, J.P., Ebel, J.P., and Falcoff, R. 1974, Inhibition of steroid inducible tyrosine aminotransferase by mouse and rat interferon in hepatoma tissue culture cells, FEBS Lett., 48:297.

Borden, E.C., and Ball, L.A. 1982, Interferons: biochemical cell growth inhibitory, and immunological effects, Prog. Hematol., 12:299.

Branca, A.A., and Baglioni, C. 1981, Evidence that types I and II interferons have different receptors, Nature, 294:768.

Branca, A.A., and Baglioni, C. 1982, Human interferon: binding to and degradation by a human cell line, J. Cell. Biochem. (suppl.), 6:95.

Cayley, P.J., Knight, M., and Kerr, I.M. 1982, Virus-mediated inhibition of the $ppp(A2'p)_n A$ system and its prevention by interferon, Biochem. Biophys. Res. Commun., 104:376.

Clemens, M.J., Pain, V.M., Wong, S.T., and Henshaw, E.C. 1982, Phosphorylation inhibits guanine nucleotide exhange on eukaryotic initiation factor 2, Nature, 296:93.

Clemens, M.J., and Williams, B.R.G. 1978, Inhibition of cell-free protein synthesis by $pppA2'p5'A2'p5'A$: a novel oligonucleotide synthesized by interferon-treated L cell extracts, Cell, 13:565.

Doetsch, P., Wu, J.M., Sawada, Y., and Suhadolnik, R.J. 1981, Synthesis and characterization of $(2'-5')ppp3'dA(p3'dA)_n$, an analogue of $(2'-5')pppA8pA)_n$, Nature, 291:355.

Dougherty, J.P., Samantha, H., Farrell, P.J., and Lengyel, P. 1980, Interferon, double-stranded RNA, and RNA degradation: isolation of homogeneous $pppA(2'p5'A)_{n-1}$ synthetase from Ehrlich ascites tumor cells, J. Biol. Chem., 255:3813.

Epstein, D.A., Czarniechki, C.W., Jacobsen, H., Friedman, R.M., and Panet, A. 1981, A mouse cell line, which is unprotected by interferon against lytic virus infection, lacks ribonuclease F activity, Eur. J. Biochem., 118:9.

Epstein, D.A., Torrence, P.F., and Friedman, R.M. 1980, Double-stranded RNA inhibits a phosphoprotein phosphatase present in interferon-treated cells, Proc. Natl. Acad. Sci. USA, 77:107.

Farrell, P.J., Balkow, K., Hunt, T., Jackson, R.J., and Trachsel, H. 1977, Phosphorylation of initiation factor eIF-2 and the control of reticulocyte protein synthesis, Cell, 11:187.

Fellous, M., Nir, U., Wallach, D., Merlin, G., Rubinstein, M., and Revel, M. 1982, Interferon-dependent induction of mRNA for the major histocompatibility antigens in human fibroblasts and lymphoblastoid cells, Proc. Natl. Acad. Sci. USA, 79:3082.

Fitzpatrick, F.A., and Stringfellow, D.A. 1980, Virus and interferon effects on cellular prostaglandin biosynthesis, J. Immunol., 125:431.

Fuse, A., and Kuwata, T. 1978, Inhibition of DNA synthesis and alteration of cyclic adenosine 3',5'-monophosphate levels in RSa cells by human leukocyte interferon, J. Natl. Cancer Inst., 60:1227.

Gewart, D.R., Shah, S., and Clemens, M.J. 1981, Inhibition of cell division by interferons: changes in the transport and intracellular metabolism of thymidine in human lymphoblastoid (Daudi) cells. Eur. J. Biochem., 116:487.

Golgher, R.R., Williams, B.R.G., Gilbert, C.S., Brown, R.E., and Kerr, I.M. 1980, Protein kinase activity and the natural occurrence of 2-5A in interferon-treated EMC virus-infected L-cells, Ann. N.Y. Acad. Sci., 350:448.

Gordon, J., and Minks, M.A. 1981, The interferon-renaissance: molecular aspects of induction and action, Microbiol. Rev., 45:244.

Gupta, S.L. 1979, Specific protein phosphorylation in interferon-treated uninfected and virus-infected mouse L929 cells: enhancements by double-stranded RNA, J. Virol., 29:301.

Gupta, S.L., Rubin, B.Y., and Holmes, S.L. 1981, Regulation of interferon action in human fibroblasts: transient induction of specific proteins and amplification of the antiviral response by actinomycin D, Virology, 111:331.

Holmes, S.L., and Gupta, S.L. 1982, Interferon action in human fibroblasts: induction of 2'5'-oligoadenylate synthetase in the absence of detectable protein kinase activity, Arch. Virol., 72:137.

Hovanessian, A.G., Brown, R.E., and Kerr, I.M. 1977, Synthesis of a low molecular weight inhibitor of protein synthesis with enzyme from interferon-treated cells, Nature, 268-537.

Hovanessian, A.G., Menes, E., and Montagnier, L. 1981, Lack of systematic correlation between the interferon mediated antiviral state and the levels of 2-5A synthetase and protein kinase in three different types of murine cells, J. Interferon Res., 1:179.

Hovanessian, A.G., and Riviere, Y. 1980, Interferon-mediated induction of 2-5A synthetase and protein kinase in the liver and spleen of mice infected with Newcastle disease virus or injected with poly(I) poly(C), Ann. Virol., 131E:501.

Hovanessian, A.G., Riviere, Y., Montagnier, L., Michelson, M., Lacour, J., and Lacour, F. 1982, Enhancement of interferon-mediated protein kinase in mouse and human plasma in response to treatment with polyadenylic-polyuridylic acid (Poly A:Poly U), J. Interferon Res., 2:209.

Hovanessian, A.G., Wood, J., Meurs, E., and Montagnier, L. 1979, Increased nuclease activity in cells treated with pppA2'p5'A2'p5'A, Proc. Natl. Acad. Sci. USA, 76:3261.

Illinger, D., Coupin, G., Richards, M., and Poindron, P. 1976, Rat interferon inhibits steroid-inducible glycerol 3-phosphate dehydrogenase synthesis in a rat glial cell line, FEBS Lett., 64:391.

Justesen, J., Ferbus, D., and Thang, M.N. 1980a, Elongation mechanism and substrate specificity of 2',5'-oligoadenylate synthetase, Proc. Natl. Acad. Sci. USA., 77:4618.

Justesen, J., Ferbus, D., and Thang, M.N. 1980b, 2'5' oligoadenylate synthetase, an interferon induced enzyme: direct assay methods for the products, 2'5' oligoadenylates and 2'5' co-oligonucleotides, Nucleic Acids Res., 8:3073.

Kerr, I.M., and Brown, R.E., 1978, pppA2'p5'A2'p5A: an inhibitor of protein synthesis synthesized with an enzyme fraction from interferon-treated cells, Proc. Natl. Acad. Sci. USA, 75:256.

Kerr, I.M., Brown, R.E., and Ball, L.A. 1974, Increased sensitivity of cell-free protein synthesis to double-stranded RNA after interferon treatment, Nature, 250:57.

Kimchi, A., Shulman, L., Schmidt, A., Chernajovsky, Y., Fradin, A., and Revel, M. 1979, Kinetics of the induction of three translation-regulatory enzymes by interferon, Proc. Natl. Acad. Sci. USA, 76:3208.

Kimchi, A., Shure, H., and Revel, M. 1981, Anti-mitogenic function of interferon-induced (2'-5') oligo(adenylate) and growth-related variations in enzymes that synthesize and degrade this oligonucleotide, Eur. J. Biochem., 114:5.

Knight, M., Cayley, P.J., Silverman, R.H., Wreschner, D.H., Gilbert, C.S., Brown, R.E., and Kerr, I.M. 1980, Radioimmune, radiobinding and HPLC analysis of 2-5A and related oligonucleotides from intact cells, Nature, 288:189.

Krishnamurti, C., Besancon, F., Justesen, J., Poulsen, K., and Ankel, H. 1982, Inhibition of mouse fibroblast interferon by gangliosides. Differential effects on biological activity and on induction of (2'-5') oligoadenylate synthetase, Eur. J. Biochem., 124:1.

Krishnan, I., and Baglioni, C. 1980a, Increased levels of (2'-5') oligo(A) polymerase activity in human lymphoblastoid cells treated with glucocorticoids, Proc. Natl. Acad. Sci. USA, 77:6506.

Krishnan, I., and Baglioni, C. 1980b, 2'5' oligo(A) polymerase activity in serum of mice infected with EMC virus or treated with interferon, Nature, 285:485.

Lebleu, B., Sen, G.C., Shaila, S., Cabrer, B., and Lengyel, P. 1976, Interferon, double-stranded RNA, and protein phosphorylation, Proc. Natl. Acad. Sci. USA, 73:3107.

Lengyel, P. 1982, Biochemistry of interferons and their actions, Annu. Rev. Biochem., 51:251.

Lengyel, P., Samanta, H., Dougherty, J.P., Brawner, M.E., and
    Schmidt, H. 1982, Interferons and gene activation: cloning of
    cDNA segments complementary to messenger RNA's induced by
    interferons, J. Cell Biochem. (suppl.), 6:81.
Levin, D.H., Petryshyn, R., and London, I.M. 1980, Characterization
    of double-stranded-RNA-activated kinase that phosphorylates α
    subunit of eukaryotic initiation factor 2(eIF-2α) in
    reticulocyte lysates, Proc. Natl. Acad. Sci. U.S.A., 77:832.
Lewis, J.A., Falcoff, E., and Falcoff, R. 1978, Dual action of
    double-stranded RNA in inhibiting protein synthesis in extracts
    of interferon-treated mouse L cells: translation is impaired at
    the level of initiation and by mRNA degradation, Eur. J.
    Biochem., 86:497.
Maheshwari, R.K., Banerjee, D.K., Waechter, C.J., Olden, K., and
    Friedman, R.M. 1980, Interferon treatment inhibits glycosylation
    of a viral protein, Nature, 287:454.
Mannering, G.J., Renton, K.W., el Azhary, R., and Deloria, L.B. 1980,
    Effects of interferon-inducing agents on hepatic cytochrome
    P-450 drug metabolizing systems, Ann. N.Y. Acad. Sci., 350:314.
Martin, E.M., Birdsall, N.J.M., Brown, R.E., and Kerr, I.M. 1979,
    Enzymic synthesis, characterisation and
    nuclear-magnetic-resonance spectra of pppA2'p5'A2'p5'A and
    related oligonucleotides: comparison with chemically
    synthesised material, Eur. J. Biochem., 95:295.
Matsuno, T., Shirasawa, N., and Kohno, S. 1976, Interferon suppresses
    glutamine synthetase induction in chick embryonic neural retina,
    Biochem. Biophys. Res. Commun., 70:310.
Meurs, E., Hovanessian, A.G., and Montagnier, L. 1981, Interferon
    mediated antiviral state in human MRCS cells in the absence of
    detectable levels of 2-5A synthetase and protein kinase, J.
    Interferon Res., 1:219.
Merritt, J.A., Borden, E.C., and Ball, L.A. 1982, Measurement of 2'5'
    oligoadenylate synthetase in human mononuclear cells, J. Cell
    Biochem. (suppl.), 6:97.
Minks, M.A., Benvin, S., and Baglioni, C. 1980, Mechanism of
    $pppA(2'p5'A)_n2'p5'A_{OH}$ synthesis in extracts of
    interferon-treated HeLa cells, J. Biol. Chem., 255:5031.
Minks, M.A., West, D.K., Benvin, S., and Baglioni, C. 1979,
    Structural requirements of double-stranded RNA for the
    activation of 2',5'-oligo(A) polymerase and protein kinase of
    interferon-treated HeLa cells, J. Biol. Chem., 254:10180.
Nagata, S., Mantei, N., and Weissmann, C. 1980, The structure of one
    of the eight or more distinct chromosomal genes for human
    interferon-α, Nature, 287:401.
Nebert, D.W., and Friedman, R.M. 1973, Stimulation of aryl
    hydrocarbon hydroxylase induction in cell cultures by
    interferon, J. Virol., 11:193.
Nilsen, T.W., and Baglioni, C. 1979, Mechanism for discrimination
    between viral and host mRNA in interferon-treated cells, Proc.
    Natl. Acad. Sci. U.S.A., 76:2600.

Nilsen, T.W., Maroney, P.A., and Baglioni, C. 1981, Double-stranded
    RNA causes synthesis of 2',5'-oligo(A) and degradation of
    messenger RNA in interferon-treated cells, J. Biol. Chem.,
    256:7806.
Nilsen, T.W., Maroney, P.A., Robertson, H.D., and Baglioni, C. 1982,
    Heterogeneous nuclear RNA promotes synthesis of (2',5')
    oliogadenylate and is cleaved by the (2',5')
    oligoadenylate-activated endoribonuclease, Mol. Cell Biol.,
    2:154.
Nilsen, T.W., Wood, D.L., and Baglioni, C. 1980, Virus-specific
    effects of interferon in emnryonal carcinoma cells, Nature,
    286:178.
Orchansky, P., Rubinstein, M., and Sela, I. 1982, Human interferons
    protect plants from virus infection, Proc. Natl. Acad. Sci.
    U.S.A., 79:2278.
Panet, A., Czarniecki, C.W., Falk, H., and Friedman, R.M. 1981,
    Effect of 2'5'-oligoadenylic acid on a mouse cell line partially
    resistant to interferon, Virology, 114:567.
Roberts, W.K., Hovanessian, A., Brown, R.E., Clemens, M.J., and Kerr,
    I.M. 1976, Interferon-mediated protein kinase and low-molecular-
    weight inhibitor of protein synthesis, Nature, 264-477.
Rochette-Egly, C., and Tovey, M.G. 1982, Interferon enhances
    guanylate cyclase activity in human lymphoma cells, Biochem.
    Biophys. Res. Commun., 107:150.
Samanta, H., Dougherty, J.P., and Lnegyel, P. 1980, Synthesis of
    (2'-5')(A)n from ATP: characteristics of the reaction catalyzed
    by (2'-5')(A)n synthetase purified from mouse Ehrlich ascites
    tumor cells treated with interferon, J. Biol. Chem., 255:9807.
Samuel, C.E. 1979, Mechanism of interferon action: phosphorylation
    of protein synthesis initiation factor eIF-2 in
    interferon-treated human cells by a ribosome-associated kinase
    processing site specificity similar to hemin-regulated rabbit
    reticulocyte kinase, Proc. Natl. Acad. Sci. U.S.A.., 76:600.
Schattner, A., Merlin, G., Wallach, D., Rosenberg, H., Bino, T.,
    Hahn, T., Levin, S., and Revel, M. 1981, Monitoring of
    interferon therapy by assay of (2'-5') oligo-isoadenylate
    synthetase in human peripheral white blood cells, J. Interferon
    Res., 1:587.
Schneck, J., Rager-Zisman, B., Rosen, O.M., and Bloom, B.R. 1982.
    Genetic analysis of the role of cAMP in mediating effects of
    interferon, Proc. Natl. Acad. Sci. U.S.A.., 79:1879.
Sekar, V., Atmar, V.J., Krim, M., and Kuehn, G.D. 1982, Interferon
    induction of polyamine-dependent protein kinase activity in
    Ehrlich ascites tumor cells, Biochem. Biophys. Res. Commun.,
    106:305.
Sen, G.C., Gupta, S.L., Brown, G.E., Lebleu, B., Rebello, M.A., and
    Lengyel, P. 1976, Interferon treatment of Ehrlich ascites tumor
    cells: effects on exogenous mRNA translation and tRNA
    inactivation in the cell extract, J. Virol., 17:191.

Sen, G.C., Shaila, S., Lebleu, B., Brown, G.E., Desrosiers, R.C., and Lengyel, P. 1977, Impairment of reovirus mRNA methylation in extracts of interferon-treated Ehrlich ascites tumor cells: further characteristics of the phenomenon, J. Virol., 21:69.

Sen, G.C., Taira, H., and Lengyel, P. 1978, Interferon, double-stranded RNA, and protein phosphorylation: characteristics of a double-stranded RNA-activated protein kinase system partially purified from interferon-treated Ehrlich ascites tumor cells, J. Biol. Chem., 253:5915.

Shulman, L., and Revel, M. 1980, Interferon-dependent induction of mRNA activity for (2'5')oligo-isoadenylate synthetase, Nature, 288:98.

Siegal, G.P., Thorgeirsson, U.P., Russo, R.G., Wallace, D.M., Liotta, L.A., and Berger, S.L. 1982, Interferon enhancement of the invasive capacity of Ewing sarcoma cells in vitro, Proc. Natl. Acad. Sci. U.S.A., 79:4064.

Siekierka, J., Mauser, L., and Ochoa, S. 1982, Mechanism of polypeptide chain initiation in eukaryotes and its control by phosphorylation of the α subunit of initiation factor 2, Proc. Natl. Acad. Sci. U.S.A., 79:2537.

Silverman, R.H., Cayley, P.J., Knight, M., Gilbert, C.S., and Kerr, I.M. 1982, Control of the $ppp(A2'p)nA$ system in HeLa cells. Effects of interferon and virus infection, Eur. J. Biochem., 124:131.

Silverman, R.H., Wreschner, D.H., Gilbert, C.S., and Kerr, I.M. 1981, Synthesis, characterization and properties of $ppp(A2'p)_n ApCp$ and related high-specific-activity ^{32}P-labelled derivatives of $ppp(A2'p)_n A$, Eur. J. Biochem., 115:79.

Singh, G., Renton, K.W., and Stebbing, N. 1982, Homogeneous interferon from E. coli depresses hepatic cytochrome P-450 and drug biotransformation, Biochem. Biophys. Res. Commun., 106:1256.

Slattery, E., Ghosh, N., Samanta, H., and Lengyel, P. 1979, Interferon, double-stranded RNA, and RNA degradation: activation of an endonuclease by $(2'-5')A_n$, Proc. Natl. Acad. Sci. U.S.A., 76:4778.

Sokawa, Y., Ando, T., and Ishihara, Y. 1980, Induction of 2',5'-oligoadenylate synthetase and interferon in mouse trigeminal ganglia infected with herpes simplex virus, Infect. Immunol., 28:719.

Sreevalsan, T., Rozengurt, E., Taylor-Papadimitriou, J., and Burchell, J. 1980, Differential effect of interferon on DNA synthesis: 2-deoxyglucose uptake and ornithine decarboxylase activity in 3T3 cells stimulated by polypeptide growth factors and tumor promoters, J. Cell Physiol., 104:1.

Stark, F.R., Dower, W.J., Schimke, R.T., Brown, R.E., and Kerr, I.M. 1979, 2-5A synthetase: assay, distribution and variation with growth or hormone status, Nature, 278-471.

Stewart, W.E., II, De Clercq, E., Billiau, A., Desmyter, J., and De
    Somer, P. 1972, Increased susceptibility of cells treated with
    interferon to the toxicity of polyriboinosinic
    acid.polyribocytidylic acid, Proc. Natl. Acad. Sci. U.S.A.,
    69:1851.
Williams, B.R.G., Golgher, R.R., Brown, R.E., Gilbert, C.S., and
    Kerr, I.M. 1979, Natural occurrence of 2-5A in interferon-
    treated EMC virus-infected L cells, Nature, 282:582.
Williams, B.R.G., Golgher, R.R., Hovanessian, A.G., and Kerr, I.M.
    1980, The involvement of the 2-5A(pppA2'p5'A2'p5'A) system and
    protein kinases in the antiviral and anticellular effects of
    interferon, in: "Developments in Antiviral Therapy", L.H.
    Collier and J. Oxford, eds., Academic Press, London, pp.
    173-187.
Williams, B.R.G., and Kerr, I.M. 1978, Inhibition of protein
Williams, B.R.G., Kerr, I.M., Gilbert, C.S., White, C.N., and Ball,
    L.A. 1978, Synthesis and breakdown of pppA2'p5'A2'p5'A and
    transient inhibition of protien synthesis in extracts from
    interferon-treated and control cells, Eur. J. Biochem., 92:455.
Williams, B.R.G., and Read, S.E. 1981, Detection of elevated levels
    of interferon-induced 2-5A synthetase in infectious diseases and
    on parturition, in: "Proceedings of the Biology of the
    Interferon System", E. De Maeyer, G. Galasso, and H.
    Schellekens, eds., Elsevier, New York, pp. 111-114.
Williams, B.R.G., Read, S.E., Freedman, M.H., Carver, D.H., and
    Gelfand, E.W. 1982, The assay of 2-5A synthetase as an indicator
    of interferonactivity and virus infection in vivo, in:
    "Chemistry and Biology of Interferons. Relationship to
    Therapeutics", UCLA Symposia on Molecular and Cellular Biology
    XXV, T.C. Merigan, and R.M. Friedman, eds., Academic Press, New
    York.
Wood, J.N., and Hovanessian, A.G. 1979, Interferon enhances 2-5A
    synthetase in embryonal carcinoma cells, Nature, 282, 74.
Wreschner, D.H., McCauley, J.W., Skehel, J.J., and Kerr, I.M. 1981,
    Interferon action--sequence specificity of the ppp(A2'p)n-
    dependent ribonuclease, Nature, 289:414.
Wreschner, D.H., Silverman, R.H., James, T.C., Gilbert, C.S., and
    Kerr, I.M. 1982, Affinity labelling and characterisation of the
    ppp(A2'p)nA-dependent endoribonuclease from different mammalian
    sources, Eur. J. Biochem., in press.
Yaron, M., Yaron, I., Gurari-Rotman, D., Revel, M., Lindner, H.R.,
    and Zor, U. 1977, Stimulation of prostaglandin E production in
    culture human fibroblasts by poly(I)ˑpoly(C) and human
    interferon, Nature, 267:457.
Zilberstein, A., Kimchi, A., Schmidt, A., and Revel, M. 1978,
    Isolation of two interferon-induced translational inhibitors: a
    protein kinase and an oligo-isoadenylate synthetase, Proc. Natl.
    Acad. Sci. USA, 75:4734.

IMMUNOLOGICAL ACTIONS

ANNAPURNA VYAKARNAM

Ludwig Institute for Cancer Research, MRC Centre
Hills Road, Cambridge, England, CB2 2QH

Interferons were originally discovered for their ability to interfere with viral replication and were long thought to be primarily antiviral agents. The possibility that they could play a non-antiviral role came first from studies in which it was demonstrated that interferon could enhance the killing of tumor cells by normal lymphocytes both in vitro and in vivo. Initially such studies were carried out with virus induced tumors, where it was shown that interferon preparations could interfere with the process of transformation and the production of tumors by oncogenic viruses (for review see, Gresser and Tovey, 1978). Subsequently such studies were carried out with chemically induced tumors demonstrating the ability of interferon to affect the proliferation of tumor cells with no viral aetiology. However the view that interferon could affect host cell metabolism and function was held with some scepticism due to contaminating substances in interferon preparations. Better purification techniques then became available and it was possible to demonstrate that the purified preparations retained similar activities as the crude material. Using purified preparations, it is now clear from several in vitro and in vivo studies that interferons are capable of affecting a wide range of cell functions which includes their ability to both enhance and inhibit various immune responses (Gresser, 1977; Balkwill, 1979; Gresser, 1980).

INTERACTION OF IFN WITH THE IMMUNE SYSTEM

Interferons are produced in the course of various immune reactions. Typically γ interferon is produced by T and B lymphocytes, in collaboration with macrophages, in response to a variety of soluble antigens, mitogens and allogeneic cells. The

requirement for such cells to interact with macrophages depends on
the type of inducing agent. α interferon is produced by a wide range
of cells including lymphocytes, macrophages and cells infected with
viruses and can be induced by several intracellular microorganisms,
products of bacteria and inducing agents such as double stranded RNA.
With the development of antisera to the various interferons it has
become clear that a given inducing agent can induce more than one
type of interferon and that a given cell is capable of producing more
than one class of interferon (Vengris et al., 1975).

The interaction of interferons with the cells of the immune
system occurs via specific receptors on the cell membrane as
demonstrated by the ability of anti-interferon sera to block such
interactions and forms a first step in their ability to affect cell
function. Recent reports have indicated that α and β interferons
share common receptors which are distinct from the receptors for γ
interferon.

Most of the data considering the immunomodulating effects of
interferon have been carried out with the well characterized α and β
interferons both in mice and humans. Some of the cells of the immune
system with which they interact are considered below.

EFFECTS OF IFN ON B CELLS

In vivo and in vitro studies have demonstrated that the
injection of interferon before antigen administration enhances
antibody production while its injection after antigen administration
suppresses such responses. Furthermore high doses of interferon have
been shown to inhibit in vivo plaque forming cell responses while low
doses enhanced plaque formation. These effects of interferons on IgM
and IgG antibody responses have been studied with a variety of
antigenic determinants including those to T dependent antigens such
as sheep red blood cells (SRBC) and to T independent antigens such as
the lipopolysaccharides of Salmonella typhimurium and E. coli.
Effects of interferon on IgE responses have been demonstrated by Ngan
et al. (1976) who showed that sensitized mouse spleen cells which
synthesized IgE and caused cutaneous anaphylaxis on rat skin were
prevented from doing so when incubated with interferon before
transfer. On the other hand interferon preparations have been shown
to enhance IgE-mediated histamine release from human peripheral blood
cells in vitro (Hernandez-Asensio et al., 1979).

Interferons have been shown to affect antibody responses in mice
injected with viruses. For example the response of mice infected
with murine hepatitis virus-3 to an injection of SRBC correlated with
circulating interferon levels in such animals (Virelizier et al.,
1976). The presence of interferon before antigen administration
reduced antibody responses while its presence after antigen injection
enhanced such responses.

There is some evidence to suggest a role for IFN-γ in the regulation of B cell response by enhancing T suppressor cell function. The ability of T cell mitogens such as PHA and CON-A to inhibit antibody production in vitro has been correlated to their ability to produce γ interferon and agents which blocked the production of mitogen induced interferon also interfered with the suppressor state in an in vitro murine immune system (Johnson et al., 1977).

Interferons are thus capable of regulating antibody responses possibly by directly affecting B cells themselves as suggested by their ability to affect antibody responses to T independent antigens and by affecting the cells which can regulate B cell function.

EFFECTS OF IFN ON T CELLS

The majority of studies on the effects of interferon on T cells have been related to its effects on the development of delayed-type hypersensitivity (DTH). De Maeyer et al. (1975) reported that the injection of interferon or interferon inducers in sensitized animals prior to the inoculation of the sensitizing antigen inhibited a DTH response to it. These investigators also demonstrated that both the afferent and efferent arcs of the DTH response were inhibited by interferon in that animals injected with interferon two days prior to sensitization also had decreased DTH responses. Such studies have been carried out with haptens (e.g. picryl chloride); T dependent antigens (e.g. SRBC) and viruses (e.g. Newcastle Disease Virus) with similar results. While interferons markedly inhibit DTH responses their effects on transplantation immunity or graft survival is conflicting. This has been attributed to factors such as dosage and route of administration (Skurkovich et al., 1973; Cerottini et al., 1973; O'Reilly et al., 1976).

Although interferon has a marked inhibitory effect on the production of DTH reactions, interferon preparations have been shown to have remarkable enhancing properties on the effector cells of cell-mediated reactions. For example mouse L cell interferon markedly enhanced the cytotoxicity of sensitized murine lymphocytes for allogeneic cells in vitro (Lindahl et al., 1972). In the human system although interferon preparations have been shown to inhibit the mixed lymphocyte reaction (MLR), the sensitized cells from an MLR had greatly increased cytotoxic potential (Heron et al., 1976).

Interferons have variable effects on the different subclasses of T cells. Effector cells such as T cytotoxic cells are enhanced by it while DTH cells are inhibited. The effects of interferon on regulatory T cells such as T helper cells are not known. However it is clear that they can enhance T suppressor cell function thereby affecting a range of cell functions.

EFFECTS ON NATURAL KILLER (NK) CELLS

Natural killer cells are defined by their ability to kill a
variety of tumor and virus infected cells without the need for prior
sensitization or immunization against such targets. These effector
cells do not fall into the categories of either T or B cells as
studied by conventional cell separation techniques and are therefore
termed natural killer cells. Because of their spontaneous ability to
kill particular tumor targets, NK cells are believed to be an
important defence mechanism against tumors. It is now quite clear
from several studies that interferons play a central role in the
regulation of NK cells. NK cells are themselves capable of producing
interferon and a wide variety of interferon inducers such as poly
I-C, C.parvum, BCG and pyran co-polymer have been shown to stimulate
NK activity in mice. Furthermore interferon activity can also be
induced by bringing into contact human leukocytes and several tumor
derived tissue culture cell lines. Because of the central role of
interferon in NK regulation and the importance of such cells in
immunosurveillance, the subject of interferon regulation of NK cells
has received considerable attention (Saksela, 1981; Gresser, 1977).

Augmentation of NK Activity

Several studies both in mice and man have shown that interferon
can boost NK cell function. In mice for example it has been shown
that the administration of interferon increased the NK-mediated
cytotoxicity of peritoneal exudate, spleen and blood cells against NK
sensitive targets (Gidland et al., 1978; Herberman et al., 1979). In
the human system the treatment of peripheral blood cells with
interferon has been shown to considerably increase their NK activity
(Einhorn et al., 1978). Similarly the administration of interferon
in healthy volunteers as well as cancer patients have been shown to
increase their circulating NK levels (Einhorn, 1980), the increased
levels of such cells falling soon after cessation of the injections.
In vitro studies of cytotoxicity against human tumors has shown that
the incubation of patients lymphocytes with interferon increases
their cytotoxic potential against allogeneic tumor cells which has
been shown to be NK mediated (Varkas et al., 1980). Although the
exact mechanism of interferon mediated augmentation of NK activity is
not clear, in vitro limiting dilution experiments would suggest that
interferon augments NK function by increasing the number of active
cells as opposed to increasing the lytic potential of any one cell.
Furthermore IFN has been shown to activate pre-NK cells in the human
system and the recruitment of such cells could result in the
augmentation of NK activity (Saksela et al., 1979).

Effects of Interferon on NK Targets

Interferon can interact with target cells and alter their
reaction to the cytotoxic activity of NK cells (Trinchieri et al.,

1978). In general the effects of such interaction has been to
protect the target cells from NK-mediated cytotoxic damage. Both
tumor and normal cells have been shown to be subject to such
regulation. In the case of tumor cells IFN-mediated protection of
targets depends on the expression of specific receptors for
interferon. In particular, undifferentiated F-9 teratocarcinoma
cells which do not express interferon receptors could not be
protected whereas more differentiated teratocarcinoma lines with
interferon receptors showed good protection (Welsh et al., 1981).
The interaction of the effector cells with their targets decreases
the cytotoxic potential of the effector cells. Only those cells
which are not capable of inducing interferon are subject to such
regulation. Normal cells such as diploid fetal fibroblasts which are
sensitive to NK killing do not induce interferon and this could be
one method by which they are protected from NK attack in vivo
(Trinchieri et al., 1978).

Effects of IFN on NK Suppressor Cells

Human and mouse NK cells have been shown to be subject to
regulation by suppressor cells which belong to the monocyte-
macrophage lineage (Santoni et al., 1980; Mantovani et al., 1980).
It has been suggested that soluble factors, in particular
prostaglandins, could be the active molecule mediating such
suppression (Brunda et al., 1980). As interferon has been shown to
enhance phagocytosis and other macrophage functions it is possible
that they could lead to suppression of NK cells via the activation of
macrophages. Some indirect evidence supporting this suggestion comes
from the observation that the injection of interferon into either
healthy volunteers or patients could lead to a temporary drop in NK
activity at four to six hr post injection. As this drop is
accompanied by a maximal fever response and as prostaglandins are
known to be involved in fever responses this could be one example of
interferon mediated suppression of NK cells (Kariniemi, et al.,
1980). Such a pathway could be an important method of shutting off
NK lysis thus acting as a negative feed-back link in the regulation
of NK activity. Furthermore, in humans a subclass of T cells (T Gl
cells) characterized by having receptors for the Fc portion of IgG
(Ig population) have been shown to suppress NK cells and interferon
pretreatment of such cells has been shown to completely abrogate
their suppressive capacity. This could be an additional method by
which interferon could regulate NK function.

EFFECTS OF IFN ON MACROPHAGES

Several studies have indicated that the treatment of peritoneal
exudate cells with interferon or interferon inducers could enhance
their spreading on glass and their phagocyte potential (Rabinovitch
et al., 1977). Other effects include the ability of interferons to

enhance both the production of lysosomal enzymes by macrophages and their tumoricidal properties (Mantovani et al., 1980; Schultz et al., 1977). In addition interferon could affect macrophage function by altering the expression of their surface HLA-DR antigens. Recent reports have shown that the treatment of human peripheral blood monocytes with interferon augmented the expression of DR antigens on such cells (Rhodes and Stokes, 1982).

IFN AS A HORMONE OR LYMPHOKINE

The central role played by interferon in immune regulation and its ability to affect a wide range of cell functions has prompted several workers to describe interferon as a hormone or lymphokine. Few attempts have however been made to study the relationship between hormones and interferons. Several features distinguish interferons from hormones and these include the ability of interferon to affect viral replication and that, in general, interferons inhibit rather than stimulate cell multiplication unlike most hormones which stimulate cell growth.

Considerable efforts have been made to study the relationship between interferons and lymphokines. Lymphokines are soluble products released by antigen activated lymphocytes and include factors which can affect macrophage function and helper and suppressor factors which can affect B cells and certain subpopulation of T lymphocytes. Several attempts have been made to compare interferons with macrophage inhibition factors (MIF) which is one of the best characterized lymphokines (Bigazzi, 1979). Cell super-natants of virus infected non-lymphoid cells have been shown to contain both interferon like activity in their ability to affect viral replication, and lymphokine, in particular MIF like activity in their ability to affect macrophage migrations (Ward et al., 1972). Hence studies have concentrated on analyzing the relationship between interferons, non-lymphocyte derived MIF, and lymphocyte derived MIF (see Table I).

The results of such studies suggest that interferons as defined by their antiviral activities appear to be quite distinct from lymphokine like activities in the same culture supernatants. However the exact relationship between interferons and lymphokines depends on purifying interferon molecules to homogeneity and then studying their antiviral and lymphokine properties. It would be particularly interesting to study the lymphokine like properties of IFN-γ which is believed to be a more potent antitumor, immunoregulatory and antiviral substance than IFN α and β (de Ley et al., 1980). The ability to purify interferons by gene cloning has opened the door to a better understanding of the nature of interferons as biological mediators and the results of studies in which such purified materials are being used is awaited.

TABLE I

Major Distinctions Between Non-Lymphocyte Derived MIF and IFN

	Lymphocyte-derived MIF	Non-lymphocyte MIF	IFN
Resistance to heat	Resistant	Resistant	Not resistant
Species specificity	Not specific	Not specific	Specific except for some reports showing that IFN-γ can cross the species barrier.
Time of appearance in cultures of chick embryos infected with Mumps/Newcastle Disease Virus	Early	Early	Late
Binding of antiserum to lymphocyte derived MIF	Binds	Binds	No binding
Effect of SV40 induced MIF on in vivo DTH in mice	Suppression	Suppression	No effect

ROLE OF INTERFERONS IN DISEASE

Perhaps one of the most important non-antiviral roles that interferon has been shown to play is its ability to inhibit tumor cell growth in several animal and human studies and hence its possible use as an antitumor reagent. Although the effectiveness of interferon therapy in humans is still contentious there have been several encouraging reports in its ability to prolong the interval between recurrence of disease and the surgical removal of several tumor types. There are several possible mechanisms by which interferons could interfere with tumor cell growth in vivo, which

include its various effects on lymphoid cells and monocytes. Of
these the ability of interferons to augment in vivo NK function has
received great attention. Several attempts have been made to follow
the effects of interferon on NK cells in patients receiving
interferon therapy. In general the results of such studies have
shown an enhancement in the lymphocyte populations from such patients
to kill NK sensitive targets in vitro. However, the validity of such
observations have been questioned due to the great variations in the
ability of cells from healthy donors to kill such targets. It has
been reported for example that NK cells are affected by such factors
as age, sex, exercise (Pross and Baines, 1982). One problem has
therefore been one of defining the base line NK activity. Another
problem encountered in such studies relates to impurities in
interferon preparations used for clinical trials which could have
effects on NK function. The third problem lies in the inherent
heterogeneity of the population which mediates the killing of NK
sensitive targets in vitro and to gaps in the knowledge of the nature
of the molecules on such targets which are recognized by NK cells
(Fast et al., 1981; Timonen et al., 1981). Recent studies have
indicated that it is possible to clone human and mouse NK cells with
the help of the T cell growth factor: Interleukin II (Dennert, 1980;
Kornbluth et al., 1982). The availability of such cell lines
together with studies using gene cloned interferon preparations may
help clarify the role of interferons in metastatic disease and its
effect on NK function in such patients.

The break-down of the interferon mediated regulation of NK
activity has been suggested to be a possible cause of various
auto-immune diseases. The inability to protect normal cells against
NK attack or the ability of interferon to inhibit T cell suppressor
function has been implicated in patients with rheumatoid arthritis,
systemic lupus erythromatosis, dermatomyositis, and scleroderma
(Hooks et al., 1980). In animal models it has been shown by Gresser
et al. (1980) that new born mice and rats on receiving high doses of
interferon developed liver necrosis and were inhibited in growth. It
has been suggested that this could be due to the lack of expression
of interferon receptors by the undifferentiated stem cells which
could then be subject to attack by NK cells. This could also explain
the rapid occurence of auto immune disease in New Zealand black mice
following the administration of interferon in such animals (Heremans
et al., 1978).

The ability of NK cells to release interferon on coming in
contact with virus infected cells could help in preventing the spread
of the virus-carrier state. For example there has been a report of
impaired NK function of blood lymphocytes in patients with multiple
sclerosis (MS). As MS may be caused by a gradual increase in the
number of virus infected cells over a prolonged period of time it
could well be that the impairment in NK function in such patients
could aid the virus-carrier state (Bloom, 1980). Recently there has
been a report of improvement in the condition of such patients
receiving interferon therapy (Jacobs et al., 1981).

From the various reports it would appear that interferons have evolved as a highly conserved and an important natural defence mechanism against several viruses and tumors. However the evidence for their therapeutic role in various diseases have so far been suggestive and more direct evidence depends on further studies which look specifically at the effects of homogenous IFN preparations on defined cell populations and perhaps the definition of genetic markers linking disease states with defects in interferon production or expression.

REFERENCES

Balkwill, F.R. 1979, Interferons as cell-regulatory molecules, Cancer Immunol. Immunother., 7:7.
Bigazzi, P.E. 1979, In: "The Biology of Lymphokines" (Ed. S. Cohen, E. Pick and J.J. Oppenheim, pp243, J. Wiley, New York.
Bloom, B.R. 1980, Interferons and the immune system, Nature., 284:593.
Brunda, M.J., Herberman, R.B. and Holden, H.T. 1980, Inhibition of murine natural killer cell activity by prostaglandins, J. Immunol., 124:2682.
Cerottini, J.C., Brunner, K.T., Lindhal, P., and Gresser, I. 1973, Inhibitory effect of interferon preparation and inducers on the multiplication of transplanted allogeneic spleen cells and syngeneic bone marrow cells, Nature New Biol., 242 (118):152.
de Ley, M., van Damme, J., Claeys, H., Heine, J.W. et al 1980, Interferon induced in human leukocytes by mitogens: production, partial purification and characterization, Eur. J. Immunol., 10:877.
Dennert, G. 1980, Cloned lines of natural killer cells, Nature, 287:47.
De Maeyer, E., DeMaeyer-Grignard, J., and Vandeputte, M. 1975, Inhibition by interferon of delayed-type hypersensitivity in the mouse, Proc. Natl. Acad. Sci. U.S.A., 72:1753.
Einhorn, S., Blomgren, H., and Strander, H. 1978, Interferon and spontaneous cytotoxicity in man. I. Enhancement of the spontaneous cytotoxicity of peripheral lymphocytes by human leukocyte interferon, Int. J. Cancer, 22:405.
Einhorn, S. 1980, In "Natural cell-mediated immunity against tumours" (Ed. R.B. Herberman) p.529, Academic Press, New York.
Fast, L.D., Hansen, J.A., and Newman, W. 1981, Evidence for T-cell nature and heterogeneity within natural killer (NK) and antibody-dependent cellular cytotoxicity (ADCC) effectors: a comparison with cytolytic T lymphocytes (CTL), J. Immunol., 127:569.
Gidland, M., Orn, A., Wigzell, H., Senik, A. and Gresser, I. 1978, Enhanced NK cell activity in mice injected with interferon and interferon inducers, Nature., 273:759.

Gresser, I. 1977, On the varied biologic effects of interferon, Cell, Immunol., 34:406.

Gresser, I., and Tovey, M.G. 1978, Anti-tumor effects of interferon, Biochim. Biophys. Acta, 516:231.

Gresser, I 1980, IFN and the immune system. In: Progress in Immunology iv (Ed. M. Fougerean and J. Dausset) p. 710 Academic Press London.

Herberman, R.B., Ortaldo, J.R., and Bonnard, G.D. 1979, Augmentation by interferon of human natural and antibody-dependant cell-mediated cytotoxicity, Nature, Lond., 277:221.

Heremans, H., Billiau, A., Colombatti, A., Hilgers, J. and de Somer, P. 1978, Interferon Treatment of NZB Mice: Accelerated progression of autoimmune disease, Infect. Immunol. 21:925.

Hernandez-Asensio, M., Hooks, J.J., Ida, S., Siraganian, R., and Notkins, A.L. 1979, Interferon-induced enhancement of IgE-mediated histamine release from human basophils requires RNA synthesis, J. Immunol, 122:1601.

Heron, I., Berg, K., Cantell, K. 1976, Regulatory effect of interferon on T cells in vitro, J. Immunol., 117:1370.

Hooks, J.J., Moutsopoulos, H.M. and Notkins, A.L. 1980, The role of interferon in immediate hypersensitivity and autoimmune diseases, Ann. N.Y. Acad. Sci., 350:21.

Jacobs, L., O'Malley, J., Freeman, R., and Ekes, R. 1981, Intrathecal interferon reduces exacerbation of Multiple Sclerosis, Science, 214:1026.

Johnson, H.M., Stanton, G.J., and Baron, S. 1977, Relative ability of mitogens to stimulate production of interferon by lymphoid cells and to induce suppression of the in-vitro immune response, Proc. Soc. Exp. Biol. Med., 154:138.

Kariniemi, A.L., Timonen, T., and Kousa, M. 1980, Effect of leucocyte interferon on natural-killer cells in healthy volunteers, Scand. J. Immunol., 12:371.

Kornbluth, J., Flomenberg, N., Dupont, B. (1982), Cell surface phenotype of a cloned line of human natural killer cells, J. Immunol., 129:2831.

Lindahl, P., Leary, P., Gresser, I. 1972, Enhancement by interferon of the specific cytotoxicity of sensitized lymphocytes, Proc. Natl. Acad. Sci. U.S.A., 69:721.

Mantovani, A., Dean, J.H., Jessels, T.R. and Herberman, R.B. 1980, Augmentation of tumouricidal activity of human monocytes and macrophages by lymphokines, Int. J. Cancer, 25:691.

Ngan, J., Lee, S.H., and Kind, L.S. 1976, Suppressive effect of Ifn on ability of mouse spleen cells synthesizing IgE to sensitise rat skin for heterologous adoptive cutaneous anaphylasis J. Immunol., 117, 1063.

O'Reilly, R.J., Everson, L.K., Emodi, G., Hansen, J., Smithwick, E.M., Grimes, E., Pahwa, S., Pahwa, R., Schwarz, S., Armstrong, D., Siegal, F.P., Gupta, S., DuPont, B. and Good, R.A. 1976, Effect of exogenous interferon in cytomegalovirus infection complicating bone narrow transplantation, Clin. Immunol. Immunopath., 6:51.

Pross, H.F., and Baines, M.G. 1982, Studies of human natural killer cells. I. In vivo parameters affecting normal cytotoxic function, Int. J. Cancer, 29:383.

Rabinovitch, M., Manejias, R.E., Russo, M., and Abbey, E.F. 1977, Increased spreading of macrophages from mice treated with interferon inducers. Cell Immunol. 29:86.

Rhodes, J., and Stokes, P. 1982, Interferon-induced changes in the monocyte membrane: inhibition by retinol and retinoic acid, Immunol. 45:

Santoni, A., Riccardi, C., Barlozzari, T., and Herberman, R.B. 1980, Suppression of activity of mouse natural killer (NK) cells by activated macrophages from mice treated with pyran copolymer, Int. J. Cancer, 26:837.

Saksela, E. 1981, "Natural Killer Cells" in "Interferon 3" (Ed. Gresser, I.), Academic Press, New York. p. 45.

Schultz, R.M., Papamatheakis, J.D., and Chingos, M.A, 1977, Interferon: an inducer of macrophage activation by polyanions, Science, 197:674.

Skurkovich, S.V., Klinovaza, E.G., Alexandrovskia, I.M., Levina, N.V. and Arkhipova, N.A. 1973, Stimulation of transplantation immunity and plasma cell reaction by IFN in mice, Immunol. 25:317.

Timonen, T., Ortaldo, J.R., and Herberman, R.B. 1981, Characteristics of human large granular lymphocytes and relationship to natural killer and K cells, J. exp. Med., 153:569.

Trinchieri, G., Santoli, D., Dee, R.R., and Knowles, B. 1978, Antiviral activity induced by culturing lymphocytes with tumour derived or virus-transformed cells. Identification of the antiviral activity as interferon and characterization of the human effector cell population, J. Exp. Med., 147:1299.

Varkas, B., Vanky, T., Argov, S.A., Einhorn, S.A., and Klein, E. 1980, Role of Alloantigens in natural killing. Allogeneic but not autologous tumour biopsy cells are sensitive for interferon-induced cytotoxicity of human blood lymphocytes, J. Exp. Med. Vol. 151, pp1151.

Vengris, V.C., Stollar, B.D., Pitha, P.M. 1975, Interferon Externalization by Producing cell before induction of antiviral state, Virology, 65:410.

Virelizier, J.L., Virelizier, A.M., and Allison, A.C. 1976, Role of circulating interferon in modifications of immune reponsiveness by mouse hepatitis virus (MHV-3), J. Immunol, 117:784.

Ward, P.A., Cohen, S., and Flanagan, T.D. 1972, Leukotactic factors elaborated by virus-infected tissues, J. Exp. Med. 135:1095.

Welsh, R.M., Karre, K., Hansson, M., Kunkel, L.A., and Kiessling, K.W. 1981, Interferon-mediated protection of normal and tumour target cells against lysis by mouse natural killer cells, . Immunol., 126:219.

THE ANTITUMOR EFFECTS OF INTERFERON IN MICE

ION GRESSER

Institut de Recherches Scientifiques sur le Cancer
Laboratory of Viral Oncology, Villejuif, France

INTRODUCTION

This article will review the antitumor effects of interferon in experimental animals (more detailed reviews were published in 1972 and 1977) (Gresser, 1972; Gresser, 1977). I must state at the outset what I hope to review, and what I will intentionally omit. This article will not deal with the effects of interferon on the development of viral induced tumors (i.e. Rous virus induced sarcoma, Friend and Rauscher leukemias in mice etc.) since interferon may be acting in these systems by inhibiting viral multiplication rather than as an antitumour substance <u>per se</u>. I will assume that there are instances in which tumor growth is independent of any viral activity and that inhibition of tumor growth by interferon is mediated by mechanisms other than its antiviral activity. I will be concerned therefore with the inhibitory effects of interferon on the growth of transplantable tumors. I will discuss only work in which interferon was administered to experimental animals, and not discuss the effects of interferon inducers since these may exert multiple biologic effects which are not necessarily mediated by interferon (Gresser et al., 1978; Vignaux and Gresser, 1981).

For some years the relative impurity of the interferon preparations used raised some question as to the nature of the antitumor substance in these preparations. The finding that highly purified mouse interferon (De Maeyer-Guignard et al., 1978) (homogenous on polyacrylamide gels in SDS) exhibited the same antitumor activity in mice as the initial partially purified preparations (and that the non-interferon contaminating proteins were ineffective) has demonstrated beyond any reasonable doubt that interferon itself can exert an antitumor activity (Gresser et al.,

65

1979). However, highly purified mouse interferon is not readily
available in sufficient quantity in most laboratories, so that most
experiments are still undertaken with crude or partially purified
interferon.

Lastly, most articles deal with the inhibitory effect of
interferon on the growth of tumors. Interferon exerts a wide range
of biologic effects on cells and it may well be that in some
instances interferon may even enhance tumor growth. Thus, in one
study, pretreatment of mice with a single dose of poly I:C or 10^6
units of interferon resulted in an increase in the growth of LSTRA
tumor cells injected subcutaneously (Gazdar et al., 1973). Ryd and
co-workers (1979) reported that "the same dose of interferon that
suppressed the growth of ascites tumors, enhanced growth of
subcutaneous tumors and in one case increased the frequency of
pulmonary metastases". I will however treat these reports as
exceptions to the rule and proceed with the assumption that under
most conditions, interferon inhibits tumor growth.

THE ANTITUMOR EFFECTS OF MOUSE INTERFERON α/β

The vast majority of the work on the antitumor effects of
interferon has been done in mice. Partially purified interferon α/β
preparations were shown to inhibit the growth of transplantable
tumors of diverse origins (viral induced, induced by chemical
carcinogens or spontaneously appearing); injected intraperitoneally
(i.p.) or subcutaneously (s.c.); in allogeneic or syngeneic mouse
systems (Gresser and Bourali, 1973; Rossi et al., 1975; Bart et al.,
1980). Transplantable tumor cells multiply rapidly and usually kill
all the mice in the weeks following tumor inoculation. These are
therefore highly artificial experimental systems, when compared with
the evolution of autochthonous tumors in patients. Nevertheless
these studies have demonstrated that interferon does exert an
antitumor activity and there may be several points of interest for
clinicians which can be summarized as follows:

(a) Interferon has proven most effective when injected
repeatedly after tumor inoculation and during the period of tumor
growth. Interferon administration limited to a few injections or to
a period prior to tumor inoculation was usually ineffective.

(b) The efficacy of interferon seems to be related to the tumor
load. If the tumor load is not overwhelming, interferon treatment
can effect cures (Gresser and Bourali, 1970; Chirigos and Pearson,
1973). For example, the mean survival time of untreated mice
inoculated i.p. with ten Ehrlich ascites cells (equivalent to
approximately 5000 LD) was 18 days, and all mice were dead by the
60th day. In mice treated with interferon (treatment beginning 24 hr

after tumor inoculation and continued daily for one month); all mice
were alive by the 30th day and 90% survived beyond the sixth month.
The tumor does not appear to develop in interferon treated mice or
grows poorly for a few days and the tumor cells are then destroyed
(Gresser and Bourali, 1970).

(c) In our experience and in the experience of others (Takeyama
et al., 1978) the extent of the inhibitory effect has been roughly
proportional to the amount of interferon injected per dose.
Likewise, for a given dose of interferon daily injections afforded a
greater effect than three injections per week which was more
effective than the total amount given as one injection per week
(unpublished data). We have never observed a decrease in the
antitumor effect by increasing the dose of interferon, though this
was reported in one study on the effect of interferon on the
evolution of the "spontaneous" lymphoma of AKR mice (Bekesi et al.,
1976).

(d) Interferon administered i.p. or s.c. has inhibited the
development of both ascitic and solid tumors and has been shown to
inhibit pulmonary metastases in mice injected with tumor cells s.c.
or i.v. (Gresser and Bourali-Maury, 1972; Glasgow and Kern, 1981).
In general, it has been easier to inhibit the growth of ascitic
tumors by injecting interferon i.p., than by injection of interferon
into solid tumors implanted s.c., but we are beginning to see all
sorts of variations so that it is hard to generalize. We still have
the impression that maximal antitumor effects are observed when
direct contact between tumor cells and interferon is maximal.

(e) In most systems described to date, interferon inhibits tumor
growth, but regression of established tumors has not been reported.
This may reflect, however, the dose of interferon used, the route and
the type of tumor injected. Some preliminary work from our
laboratory suggests in fact that interferon can under some
circumstances induce regression of an established transplantable
tumor.

COMPARISONS OF THE ANTITUMOR EFFECTS OF MOUSE INTERFERON α/β WITH
MOUSE INTERFERON γ

Salvin and his co-workers (1975) were the first to suggest that
a lymphokine rich serum containing type II interferon exerted a
greater antitumor effect than serum containing an equivalent quantity
of type I interferon. They produced the type II interferon (γ) in
mice by first injecting them i.v. with mycobacterium bovis (strain
BCG) and three weeks later inoculating them i.v. with old tuberculin.
The sera of these mice contained in addition to type II interferon,
high titers of migration inhibitory factor, and "bacteriostatic,
mycostatic and hematopoiesis inhibiting activities".

A transplantable 3-methylcholanthrene-induced sarcoma was implanted s.c. and unpurified mouse sera containing either 300 units of type I or type II interferon was injected locally. Injection of type I interferon proved ineffective whereas injection of serum containing type II interferon "inhibited cell tumor growth by 97%" (Salvin et al., 1975).

Using similar methods for the production of type II interferon, Crane et al. compared the dose/response relationship for the anti-tumor activities of types I and II serum interferon injected s.c. at the site of tumor implantation (Crane et al., 1978). A marked tumor inhibitory activity was observed with both preparations but treatment with sera containing 600 units of type II interferon appeared "strikingly more effective than 600 units of type I interferon" and roughly equivalent to about 60,000 units of type I interferon.

These two studies suggested that mouse interferon γ might exert a greater antitumor activity than interferon α/β. However, as the authors point out, no attempt was made to purify the type II interferon and the sera contained other lymphokines. Lymphokine containing sera have been shown to inhibit the growth of other transplantable tumors in mice (Mouton and Daniels, 1980; Evans, 1982) and have even been reported to induce regression of localized neoplastic lesions in man (Klein et al., 1981). Since none of these lymphokines has been purified and tested individually in a given system, it is impossible to determine what part of the antitumor activity may be ascribed to interferon γ and what part to other lymphokines. These "other lymphokines" may also have exerted a synergistic/additive effect. Fleischmann et al. (1980) have reported that crude type II interferon can potentiate the antitumor effect of type I interferon.) Meaningful comparisons between interferons in terms of a given biologic activity - i.e. antitumor/antiviral - will have to be expressed in terms of molar ratios rather than in terms of another biologic activity (i.e. antiviral units) as is currently practiced.

Lastly, a given interferon (or species of interferon) may be more effective than another interferon in one tumor system but less effective in a different tumor system or by a different route of injection. Thus, although it may turn out that interferon γ does exert a more potent antitumor activity more often than interferon α or interferon β, there is just not adequate data at present to take any position.

COMBINATION THERAPY

Since combination chemotherapy has generally proven more effective than single drug therapy, it was logical to combine interferon therapy with other antitumor treatments. Chirigos and

Pearson (1973) found that reduction of a transplantable tumor in mice by BCNU prior to interferon treatment resulted in 72% cure rate compared to a 25% cure rate for BCNU alone and 0% for interferon alone.

In our experience daily administration of interferon initiated after clinical diagnosis of the "spontaneously" appearing lymphoma in AKR mice resulted in an increased average survival of 100% (Gresser et al., 1976). When the tumor mass was first reduced by cyclophosphamide, interferon therapy increased survival time by about 200% (Gresser et al., 1978).

Relatively small amounts of mouse interferon were shown to increase to a slight degree survival in mice injected with L1210 cells treated with a combination of 6-mercaptopurine-methotrexate whereas it did not enhance the antitumor effect of 6-mercaptopurine, adriamycin, cytosine arabinoside or cyclophosphamide (Slater et al., 1981). It should be noted however that in this study none of the therapeutic regimens seemed very effective.

Other therapies coupled with interferon have included sodium butyrate (Bourgeade et al., 1979), isoprinosine (Cerutti et al., 1978) or local hyperthermia (Yerushalmi et al., 1982).

In the search for compounds capable of enhancing interferon's antitumor action, some investigators have found substances which diminish its activity. Thus, Baron and co-workers (1981) noted that trans-retinoic acid enhanced local tumor growth and partially inhibited interferon action.

Since the mechanism of the antitumor action of interferon is still unknown, all experimental combination therapy has been empirical. There is also another approach that as to my knowledge has not yet been tried, and that is to determine whether interferon treatment can render tumor cells more sensitive to chemo- or radiation therapy. Stewart and his colleagues showed (1972) that a short term incubation of mouse cells with interferon resulted in an increased sensitivity to the toxic effects of polyriboinosinic-polyribocytidylic acid. It seems possible that in a similar manner, interferon might enhance the sensitivity of tumor cells in vivo to tumorcidal drugs, monoclonal antibodies, X-irradiation, hyperthermia, etc.

EFFECT OF HUMAN AND MOUSE INTERFERON IN ATHYMIC NUDE MICE INOCULATED WITH TRANSPLANTABLE TUMORS

A variety of human tumors grow in the athymic nude mouse and several investigators have determined the effect of human interferon preparations injected either systemically or directly into the

growing tumor. Carter and his colleagues (1978) found that human
interferon β inhibited the growth of tumor cells from established
human cell lines and that the in vivo sensitivity of the cells
correlated well with their in vitro interferon sensitivity with one
interesting exception. The Daudi cell line derived from a Burkitt
lymphoma is one of the most interferon sensitive cell lines and yet
interferon did not inhibit the growth of these cells transplanted to
nude mice.

Balkwill and colleagues (1980) implanted pieces of primary
infiltrating breast carcinomas into nude mice. For two of three
tumors tested, they showed that repeated s.c. injections of human
interferon-α (Namalwa) delayed the appearance of tumors, inhibited
the number of tumors per mouse and the number of mice with tumors.
Purified human interferon-α also inhibited the growth of an
established breast carcinoma in nude mice, but did not alter tumor
morphology, cellularity or mucin production (Balkwill et al, 1980).
As discussed above, the inhibiting effect was more pronounced when
interferon was administered repeatedly. Thus, a regimen of seven
daily injections of 2×10^6 u was more effective than injections
three time per week of 4.7×10^6 u which in turn was more effective
than one injection per week of 1.4×10^7 u. By examining the effects
of human and mouse interferons on the levels of 2-5A-synthetase in
the tumor and spleen and their effects on NK cell function the
investigators concluded that human interferon was acting by
inhibiting directly the proliferation of tumor cells (Balkwill et
al., 1982). However, in the discussion of their results, they refer
to unpublished data indicating that mouse cell interferon which "has
no antiviral or cell growth inhibitory activity on human cells in
vitro, can inhibit the growth of this human tumor in nude mice".

Similar results were reported by Masuda and colleagues (1982)
who found that human leucocyte interferon (5×10^6 u/mouse) inhibited
the growth of one line of a human osteosarcoma but had little effect
on another oesteosarcoma cell line. Treatment could even be
initiated two weeks after tumor inoculation and almost completely
arrest tumor growth.

Yokota and his colleagues (1976) reported that mouse interferon,
but not human interferon inhibited the mouse sarcoma 180 transplanted
to nude mice, whereas human but not mouse interferon inhibited the
growth of human Hela cells in nude mice.

In contrast to this ensemble of results, De Clercq and his
colleagues (1978) did not observe any inhibitory effect of either
human or mouse interferon (5×10 units/kg) on the growth of two
established human tumor cell lines transplanted into nude mice,
although repeated administration of poly I·poly C which induced mouse
interferon, did inhibit tumor growth.

POSSIBLE MECHANISMS FOR THE ANTITUMOR EFFECTS OF INTERFERON

Although several possibilities may be invoked to explain the antitumor effects of interferon, there really is no clear-cut answer. There is experimental evidence to suggest that several mechanisms may be involved: a direct effect of interferon on the tumor itself and/or an indirect effect via the host. I have listed the different possibilities in Table I and have discussed these possibilities in three recent brief reviews (Gresser and Tovey, 1978; Gresser, 1982). Some of these points may however be summarized here. First, interferon can inhibit tumor cell division in vitro. Although interferon is usually not directly cytocidal, inhibition of tumor cell multiplication can be associated with cell death (Tovey and Brouty-Boyé, 1979). It is important to emphasize, however, that the inhibitory effect of interferon on tumor cell multiplication does not appear to be specific, since the division of normal cells is also inhibited (Lindahl-Magnusson et al., 1971).

Interferon can induce alterations in tumor (and normal) cells which may affect their behavior. These cells may therefore respond differently to a variety of host humoral factors or effector cells as well as to a variety of foreign substances. Since the surface of these cells is altered, transport of vital substances may be modified (Brouty-Boyé and Tovey, 1978).

Tumors secrete a variety of factors ("oncotrophins") (Gresser, 1977) which may be important in influencing the rate at which the

TABLE I
Possible Mechanisms of the Antitumor Effects of Interferon

Direct Effects of Interferon on Tumor Cells

(1) Inhibition of tumor cell multiplication
(2) Interferon induced alterations in cells which may affect their behaviour
(3) Effect of interferon on the production of factors by tumor cells
(4) Reversion of the transformed and malignant phenotype by interferon

Effects of Interferon on the Host

(1) Effector cells
(2) Antibody formation
(3) Non specific mechanisms
(4) Interaction between stroma and tumor

tumor grows, by stimulating directly tumor cell multiplication, depressing the host immune response, inducing vascularization of the tumor, etc. Interferon may inhibit or enhance the production of a variety of substances by tumor cells.

As a fourth possibility, interferon treatment of transformed cells in vitro can induce a reversion of the transformed and malignant phenotype to a more normal phenotype. For example, X-ray transformed cells passaged with interferon showed a progressive reversion of the transformed phenotype, exemplified by changes in morphology, distribution of cytoskeletal structures, saturation density and a loss of tumorigenicity (Brouty-Boyé and Gresser, 1981). It would seem of considerable interest to determine in appropriate experimental systems whether interferon treatment of a tumor bearing animal is also associated with an attenuation or reversion of the malignant phenotype.

The finding that human interferon preparations can inhibit the growth of human tumors transplanted into nude mice certainly suggests that interferon can exert an antitumor effect by affecting the tumor cells directly (Carter et al., 1978; Balkwill et al., 1980; Balkwill et al., 1982; Masuda et al., 1982; Yokota et al., 1976) (the activity of the human interferon preparations on mouse cells should have been too low to have exerted a significant effect). However, some years ago, we showed that mouse interferon protected mice inoculated with mouse lymphoma cells selected for resistance to interferon (Gresser et al., 1972; Gresser and Bourali-Maury, 1973). These results suggested to us that at least part of interferon's antitumor effect in this experimental system was host mediated.

How might interferon exert an antitumor effect via the host? Both specific cellular and humoral mechanisms have been invoked as well as non specific mechanisms, and the interaction of interferon with these mechanisms has received considerable attention. Interferon has been shown to enhance the cytotoxicity of sensitized T lymphocytes (Lindahl et al., 1972) and NK cells for tumor target cells (Saksela, 1981) and phagocytosis of tumor cells by macrophages (Gresser and Bourali, 1970). I doubt however that the antitumor effects of interferon can be explained solely by enhancement of effector cell activity.

Interferon can influence the production by host cells of prostaglandins, histamine and hormones. It may be that the enhanced release of such pharmacologically active substances also contributes to the antitumor action of interferon.

Lastly, there is the possibility that interferon may influence the micro-environment of the tumor, the interaction of the growing tumor with the surrounding stroma.

If the above discussion of the mechanisms responsible for the antitumor action of interferon seems incomplete and unsatisfactory, I believe it is because we do not know how interferon acts. It would be easy to conclude by saying that several mechanisms may be operative, depending on the tumor, the host and a variety of factors. Although this may be so, I believe that the mechanism(s) by which interferon inhibits tumor growth is not even listed in Table I. I am guessing that interferon is acting through a mechanism which has not yet occurred to us, or at least that has not yet been publicized. This would be a good thing if it were so, because it may then open the way for effective antitumor therapy.

ACKNOWLEDGEMENT

Work in the author's laboratory was supported by grants from the D.R.E.T., C.N.R.S. and I.N.S.E.R.M.

REFERENCES

Balkwill, F., Taylor-Papadimitriou, J., Fantes, K.H., and Sebesteny, A. 1980, Human lymphoblastoid interferon can inhibit the growth of human breast cancer xenografts in athymic nude mice, Eur. J. Cancer, 16:569.

Balkwill, F.R., Moodie, E.M., Freedman, V., and Fantes, K.H. 1982, Human interferon inhibits the growth of established human breast tumours in the nude mouse, Int. J. Cancer, in press.

Baron, S., Kleyn, K.M., Russell, J.K., and Blalock, J.E. 1981, Retinoid acid : Enhancement of a tumor and inhibition of interferon's antitumor action, J. Natl. Cancer Inst., 1:95.

Bart, R.S., Porzio, N.R., Kopf, A.W., Vilcek, J.T., Cheng, E.H., and Farcet, Y. 1980, Inhibition of growth of B16 murine malignant melanoma by exogenous interferon, Cancer Res., 40:614.

Bekesi, J.G., Roboz, J.P., Zimmerman, E., and Holland, J.F. 1976, Treatment of spontaneous leukemia in AKR mice with chemotherapy, immunotherapy or interferon, Cancer Res., 36:631.

Bourgeade, M-F., Cerutti, I., and Chany, C. 1979, Enhancement of interferon antitumor action by sodium butyrate, Cancer Res., 39:4720.

Brouty-Boyé, D., and Tovey, M.G. 1978, Inhibition by interferon of thymidine uptake in chemostat cultures of L1210 cells, Intervirology, 9:243.

Brouty-Boyé, D., and Gresser, I. 1981, Reversibility of the transformed and neoplastic phenotype. I. Progressive reversion of the phenotype of x-ray transformed C3H/10T1/2 cells under prolonged treatment with interferon, Int. J. Cancer, 28:165.

Carter, W.A., Leong, S.S., and Horoszewicz, J.S. 1978, Human fibroblast interferon in the control of neoplasia in: "Antiviral Mechanisms in the Control of Neoplasia," P. Chandra, ed., Plenum Press, New York and London.

Cerutti, I., Chany, C., and Schlumberger, J.F. 1978, Short
    Communication : Isoprinosine increases the anti-tumor action of
    interferon, Int. J. Immunopharmacol., 1:59.
Chirigos, M.A., and Pearson, J.W. 1973, Brief Communication : Cure
    of murine leukemia with drug and interferon treatment, J. Natl.
    Cancer Inst., Vol. 51, 4:1367.
Crane, J.L. Jr., Glasgow, L.A., Kern, E.R., and Youngner, J.S.
    1978, Inhibition of murine osteognic sarcomas by treatment with
    type I or type II interferon, J. Natl. Cancer Inst., 3:871.
De Clercq, E., Georgiades, J., Edy, V.G., and Sobis, H. 1978,
    Effect of human and mouse interferon and of polyriboinosinic
    acid. Polyribocytidylic acid on the growth of human
    fibrosarcoma and melanoma tumors in nude mice, Eur. J. Cancer,
    11:1273.
De Maeyer-Guignard, J., Tovey, M.G., Gresser, I., and
    De Maeyer, E. 1978, Purification of mouse interferon by
    sequential affinity chromatography on poly(U) and
    antibody-agarose columns, Nature, 271:622.
Evans, C.H. 1982, An immunologic hormone with anticarcinogenic and
    antitumor activity, Cancer Immunol. Immunother., 12:181.
Fleischmann, W.R. Jr., Kleyn, K.M., and Baron, S. 1980,
    Potentiation of virus-induced interferon by mouse immune
    interferon preparations, J. Natl. Cancer Inst., 5:963.
Gazdar, A.D., Sims, H., Spahn, G.J., and Baron, S. 1973,
    Interferon mediates enhancement of tumor growth and
    virus-induced sarcomas in mice, Nature New Biology, 245:77.
Glasgow, L.A., and Kern, E.R. 1981, Effect of interferon
    administration on pulmonary osteogenic sarcomas in an
    experimental murine model, J. Natl. Cancer Inst., 1:207.
Gresser, I., Bourali, C., Chouroulinkov, I., Fontaine-Brouty-Boyé,
    D., and Thomas, M-T. 1970, Treatment of neoplasia in mice with
    interferon preparations. Second Conference on Antiviral
    Substances, The New York Academy of Sciences, 173:694.
Gresser, I., and Bourali, C. 1970, Antitumor effects of interferon
    preparations in mice, J. Natl. Cancer Inst., 45:365.
Gresser, I. 1972, Antitumor effects of interferon
    in: Advances in Cancer Research," G. Klein and S. Weinhouse,
    eds., Academic Press, New York and London, 16:97.
Gresser, I., and Bourali-Maury, C. 1972, Inhibition by interferon
    preparations of the growth of a solid malignant tumor and the
    development of pulmonary metastases in mice, Nature New Biology,
    236:78.
Gresser, I., Maury, C., and Brouty-Boyé, D. 1972, On the mechanism
    of the antitumor effect of interferon in mice, Nature, 239:167.
Gresser, I., and Bourali-Maury, C. 1973, The antitumor effect of
    interferon in lymphocyte and macrophage depressed mice, Proc.
    Soc. Exp. Biol. Med., 144:896.
Gresser, I., Maury, C., and Tovey, M.G. 1976, Interferon and
    murine leukemia. VII. Therapeutic effect of interferon
    preparations after diagnosis of lymphoma in AKR mice, Int. J.
    Cancer, 17:647.

Gresser, I. 1977, Antitumor effects of interferon
    in: "Cancer - a Comprehensive Treatise," Chemotherapy,
    F. Becker, ed., Plenum Press, New York, 5:521.
Gresser, I., Maury, C., Bandu, M-T., Tovey, M.G., and
    Maunoury, M-T. 1978, Role of endogenous interferon in the
    antitumor effect of poly I˙C and statolon as demonstrated by the
    use of anti-mouse interferon serum, Int. J. Cancer, 21:72.
Gresser, I., Maury, C., and Tovey, M.G. 1978, Efficacy of combined
    interferon cyclophosphamide therapy after diagnosis of lymphoma
    in AKR mice, Eur. J. Cancer, 14:97.
Gresser, I., and Tovey, M.G. 1978, Antitumor effects of
    interferon, Biochem. Biophys. Acta, 516:231.
Gresser, I., De Maeyer-Guignard, J., Tovey, M.G., and
    De Maeyer, E. 1979, Electrophoretically pure mouse interferon
    exerts multiple biologic effects, Proc. Natl. Acad. Sci. USA,
    76:5308.
Gresser, I. 1982, How does interferon inhibit tumor growth?,
    Proceedings of the Royal Society, in press.
Klein, E., Case, R.W., Holtermann, O., Milgrom, H., Hahn, G., and
    Pfeffer, F. 1981, Clinical effects of local lymphokine
    administration on neoplastic lesions, Proc. Am. Assoc. Cancer
    Res., 22:164.
Lindahl, P., Leary, P. and Gresser, I. 1972, Enhancement by
    interferon of the specific cytotoxicity of sensitized
    lymphocytes, Proc. Natl. Acad. Sci. USA, 69:721.
Lindahl-Magnusson, P., Leary, P., and Gresser, I. 1971, Interferon
    and cell division. VI. Inhibitory effect of interferon on the
    multiplication of mouse embryo and mouse kidney cells in primary
    cultures, Proc. Soc. Exp. Biol. Med., 138:1044.
Masuda, S., Fukuma, H., and Beppu, Y. 1982, Antitumor effects of
    human leukocyte interferon on human osteosarcomas transplanted
    in nude mice, in press.
Mouton, R.G., and Daniels, J.C. 1980, Effect of
    lymphokine-containing sera on adenocarcinoma BW10232 and
    melanoma B16 in C57Bl/6 mice, J. Natl. Cancer Inst., 4:901.
Ryd, W., Hagmar, B., Lundgren, E., and Strannegärd, O. 1979,
    Discrepant effects of interferon on murine syngeneic ascites
    tumors and their solid metastasizing counterparts, Int. J.
    Cancer, 23:397.
Rossi, J.B., Marchegiani, M., Matarese, G.P., and Gresser, I.
    1975, Brief Communication : Inhibitory effect of interferon on
    multiplication of Friend Leukemia cells in vivo, J. Natl. Cancer
    Inst., 54:993.
Saksela, E. 1981, Interferon and natural killer cells
    in: "Interferon III," I. Gresser, ed., 3:45, Academic Press, New
    York and London.
Salvin, S.B., Youngner, J.S., Nishio, J., and Neta, R. 1975, Brief
    Communication : Tumor suppression by a lymphokine released into
    the circulation of mice with delayed hypersensitivity, J. Natl.
    Cancer Inst., 5:1233.

Slater, L.M., Wetzel, M.W., and Cesario, T. 1981, Combined
    interferon - Antimetabolite therapy of murine L1210 leukemia,
    Cancer, 48:5.
Stewart, W.E. II, De Clercq, E., Billiau, A., Desmyter, J. and
    De Somer, P. 1972, Increased susceptibility of cells treated
    with interferon to the toxicity of
    polyriboinosinic-polyribocytidylic acid, Proc. Natl. Acad. Sci.
    USA, 7:1851.
Takeyama, H., Kawashima, K., Kobayashi, M., Yamada, K., and
    Ito, Y. 1978, Antitumor effect of interferon preparations on
    murine transplantable tumors, Gann, 69:641.
Tovey, M.G., and Brouty-Boyé, D. 1979, The use of the chemostat to
    study the relationship between cell growth rate, viability and
    the effect of interferon on L1210 cells, Exptl. Cell Res.,
    118:383.
Vignaux, F., and Gresser, I. 1981, Hypoglycemia in mice injected
    with interferon inducers is not mediated by interferon, Inf. and
    Immun., 33:331.
Yerushalmi, A., Tovey, M.G., and Gresser, I. 1982, Antitumor
    effect of combined interferon and hyperthermia in mice, Proc.
    Soc. Exp. Biol. Med., 169:413.
Yokota, Y., Kishida, T., Esaki, K., and Kawamata, J. 1976,
    Antitumor effects of interferon on transplanted tumors in
    congenitally athymic nude mice, Biken Journal, 19:125.

LYMPHOMA

SANDRA HORNING

Department of Medicine, Division of Oncology
Stanford University Medical Center, Stanford, CA 94305

PRE-CLINICAL STUDIES

The effects of human leukocyte interferon on the proliferation
of several lymphoid cell lines have been tested (Einhorn and
Strander, 1978). A 50% reduction in cell multiplication was observed
in five of eleven Burkitt's lymphoma lines and one of two lymphocytic
lymphoma lines. Inhibition of cell multiplication in sensitive lines
occurred at interferon concentrations of 2-300 u/ml, while other
lines remained resistant at concentrations up to 10,000 u/ml. In
this system, two of two Burkitt's lines were found to be more
sensitive to leukocyte than to fibroblast interferon (Einhorn and
Strander, 1977). Additional investigation of Daudi cells, a
Burkitt's lymphoma cell line, has revealed that the antiproliferative
activity of fibroblast interferon is greatest when cells are in the
resting phase (Horoszewicz et al., 1979). However, inhibition of
growth by interferon was dose-dependent at all phases.

Sikora and colleagues prepared human-mouse hybridomas from the
neoplastic peripheral blood cells of two lymphoma patients (Sikora et
al., 1980). A dose-dependent inhibition of growth by interferon, was
observed in 14 of 17 hybrids at concentrations readily attained in
vivo. Both patients had shown clinical responses to treatment with
the same human leukocyte interferon.

Treatment of AKR mice with interferon from birth to one year
reduced the expected high incidence of spontaneous lymphomas and
increased survival time (Gresser et al., 1969). When interferon was
given after the diagnosis of lymphoma, life span was also increased.
Furthermore, some investigators have reported acute cytoreduction in
lymph nodes and spleen in mice treated with interferon (Graff et al.,
1970).

Difficulties in establishing continuous lymphoma cell lines have limited the ability to study interferon. Similarly, difficulties have been encountered with lymphoid malignancies in the tumor stem cell soft agar colony system. However, as with other neoplastic cells, the above results indicate that lymphomas are heterogeneous in their sensitivity to interferon. Sensitive cells appear to be inhibited by interferon in a dose-dependent manner. The anti-proliferative effects of interferon may vary according to the growth rate of the target and the relationship of the target to the origin of the interferon.

Additional studies with interferon in standard in vitro and animal systems may provide useful information on optimal dose and schedule for expression of antitumor effects. These may also provide insights into mechanisms of resistance and potential synergy between interferon and drug therapy. Improved understanding of the biologic response(s) integral to the antitumor effects in these systems may likewise be applicable to the human lymphomas.

CLINICAL STUDIES

Human Leukocyte Interferon

Enthusiasm for the potential clinical application of interferon in the treatment of lymphomas was generated by a case report published by Blomgren et al. (1976). A patient with stage IVB, lymphocyte-predominant Hodgkin's disease demonstrated clinical improvement in B symptoms, adenopathy and pulmonary infiltrates while receiving intramuscular interferon 5×10^6 u daily. The interferon was prepared according to the methods of Cantell by the Finnish Red Cross and had a specific activity of 10^6 reference u/mg of protein (Cantell and Hirvonen, 1978).

Merigan et al. treated six patients with non-Hodgkin's lymphoma with Cantell human leukocyte interferon, 5×10^6 u, intramuscularly, twice daily for 30 days (Merigan et al., 1978). Three of these patients had diffuse histiocytic lymphoma (DH) which was characterized by disease progression with extensive prior therapy. The other three patients had indolent, nodular lymphocytic, poorly-differentiated lymphoma (NLPD) which had been observed without treatment for at least one year. Tumor reduction was observed in each of the patients with NLPD, including a dramatic resolution of peripheral and retroperipheral lymph nodes and normalization of the bone marrow on biopsy. One patient achieved a complete remission (CR) and two patients achieved partial remissions (PR). The duration of unmaintained remissions ranged from six to 12 months. In contrast, disease progression was observed in each of the patients with DH.

These preliminary observations were followed by a report of five additional patients with nodular lymphoma, NLPD and nodular mixed lymphocytic and histiocytic (NM), treated with human leukocyte interferon in an identical manner (Louie et al., 1981). One of these patients, a man who had been heavily pretreated with multiple chemotherapeutic agents, was not evaluable for response due to early hematologic toxicity. Of the remaining four patients, two had less than 25% regression of adenopathy and two had no response. The difference in response in these reports from the same investigators using the same interferon preparation is not explained by exposure to cytotoxic therapy. Only one of the patients in the second group had received prior chemotherapy. Furthermore, a responsive patient in the initial study responded to a second course of interferon despite interval treatment with combination chemotherapy.

Gutterman et al. reported the results of treatment with interferon in 11 patients with malignant lymphoma: six with NLPD, one with DH and four with chronic lymphocytic leukemia (CLL) (Gutterman et al., 1980). The interferon used in this study was also human leukocyte interferon prepared by the Finnish Red Cross. Doses of 3 x 10^6 u (ten patients) and 9 x 10^6 u (one patient) daily IM were administered for a minimum period of four weeks. Complete or partial remissions for 18 to 46+ weeks were recorded in three of six patients with NLPD. Five of the six NLPD patients had relapsing disease and had received prior therapy. Antitumor activity was also seen in two of four patients with CLL and the single patient with DH.

The crude interferon used in these initial studies represents a pool of ten or more alpha species. The major side effects in treated patients included mild, readily reversible myelosuppression, initial fever and myalgias, anorexia and fatigue.

With this background, the American Cancer Society (ACS) sponsored the purchase of human leukocyte interferon prepared by the Finnish Red Cross for a Phase II multi-institutional study of Hodgkin's and non-Hodgkin's lymphomas. Participating institutions included Stanford University, M.D. Anderson Hospital and Tumor Institute and Memorial Sloan-Kettering Cancer Center. Non-Hodgkin's lymphomas were classified according to the modified system of Rappaport by one of three designated pathologists. Patients with nodular lymphoma had been biopsied within 60 days of randomization. Uniform staging consisted of interview and examination, bipedal lymphography and bone marrow biopsy. Eligibility requirements included measurable disease, no cytotoxic therapy with four weeks and antineoplastic therapy at least 30 days after the conclusion of interferon. Patients were initially randomized among doses of 1 x 10^6 u, 2 x 10^6 u daily for four weeks. Subsequent modifications included dropping the low and intermediate doses and allowing the use of additional interferon at the intermediate dose for patients with stable or responding disease after four weeks of 9 x 10^6 interferon daily.

Forty-nine patients were treated: 15 with NLPD, three with NM, ten with CLL or diffuse lymphocytic well-differentiated (DLWD), 11 with DH and ten with Hodgkin's disease. Antitumor activity was seen in one third of patients with the favorable, nodular subtypes NLPD and NM, particularly those without previous treatment (unpublished data). Eighty percent of the responses were seen at the 9×10^6 u dose. The majority of patients with CLL, DLWD and Hodgkin's had stable disease following interferon treatment. Disease progression was most often noted during therapy for DH, although two patients had minimal responses. With relatively small patient numbers and brief exposure to interferon, one can only conclude that limited evidence of antitumor activity (usually <50% regression of measurable disease) was observed, primarily among those patients with nodular lymphoma. Proper interpretation of these results requires consideration of histologic subtype, previous therapy and tempo of current disease as well as the dose and duration of interferon therapy. Additional undefined host and tumor characteristics are undoubtedly relevant to these observations and those that preceded them.

Recombinant Leukocyte Interferon

Leukocyte interferon clone A, produced by recombinant DNA technology, became available for clinical studies in 1981. This material differs from the human product in its greater purity. In addition it is a single species of interferon. Initial clinical testing of recombinant interferon established pharmacokinetics and toxicity similar to human interferon (Horning et al., 1982; Gutterman et al., 1982). Antitumor activity was seen in five of six nodular lymphoma patients treated in a single ascending dose study. Additional Phase I studies have also established evidence of tumor regression in patients with lymphoma, including partial responses in four with NLPD and one with DLWD treated with escalating intramuscular doses three times weekly (Sherwin et al., 1982). A Phase II study in refractory nodular lymphoma patients treated three times weekly at the maximal tolerated dose is in progress. Phase III studies in untreated patients are planned. These trials will provide efficacy data among relatively similar patients, although pertinent only to the dose and scheduled used.

Other Interferons

Other interferon preparations have been less well studied in patients with malignant lymphoma. Lymphoblastoid interferon is currently under study. Additional molecular species of leukocyte interferon are becoming available for clinical testing through recombinant DNA technology. Combinations of these interferons should become available as well. As mentioned, in vitro data suggests that leukocyte interferon may be preferable in the treatment of lymphoma (Einhorn and Strander, 1977). Thus, one or more subtypes of alpha interferon normally involved in lymphoid regulation may possess the

greatest antiproliferative activity against lymphomas. In addition
to leukocyte interferon, recombinant beta (fibroblast) and gamma
(immune) interferon are entering clinical testing.

DISCUSSION

Antiproliferative vs. Immunomodulatory Activity in Lymphoma

The antitumor activity of interferon may be direct, as it serves
to regulate cell division, or indirect in altering the host immune
system. Nodular lymphomas, in particular, may be affected by more
than one of the multiple properties interferon. Nodular lymphomas
are monoclonal B cell proliferations which may result from defects in
immune regulation. Spontaneous regressions have been noted in a
small number of patients (Krikorian et al., 1980; Gattiker et al.,
1980). Even more commonly, patients have indolent disease with
waxing and waning of their peripheral adenopathy. These
considerations lead naturally to the inference that immune modulation
by interferon may contribute to the observed antitumor effects. This
concept is especially attractive when the tumor burden is low and/or
the tempo of measurable disease suggests a more favorable interaction
between the host and the tumor.

Tests of immune function in treated lymphoma patients have
demonstrated alterations in T cell responsiveness, lymphocyte
populations and natural killer (NK) activity (Horning et al., 1982;
Rasmussen and Merigan, 1980; Huddlestone et al., 1979). To date,
these have not correlated with observed antitumor responses. Dose,
schedule and route of administration for each interferon preparation
will influence the observed immune modulation, as suggested by work
with recombinant leukocyte interferon (Maluish et al., 1982).

Future Considerations

The early investigation of interferon in malignant lymphoma was
limited by supply and cost. With the increased availability of
multiple interferon preparations, the proper design of clinical
trials and interpretation of results becomes more critical. As a
single agent interferon has shown little activity in heavily
pretreated patients with Hodgkin's disease and DH. Among patients
with nodular lymphoma, the antitumor activity of a brief pulse of
interferon is relatively weak when compared with conventional
cytotoxic therapy. However, despite high complete remission rates
with either radiotherapy or chemotherapy in advanced favorable
lymphomas, no cures are achieved. In the future, interferon may be
utilized in combination with cytotoxic therapy for induction or as an
adjuvant after cytoreduction. There is support for this approach in
that interferon is additive or synergistic in combination with
chemotherapeutic agents (Chirigos and Pearson, 1973; Gresser et al.,

1978). The potential toxicity, hematologic and nonhematologic, of this combination will require careful clinical investigation. Interferon alone may be of use in situations of low tumor burden where alteration of the immune system may allow tumor control. Another strategy might utilize interferon to enhance specific immunotherapy with other biologic response modifiers.

In order to best establish the role of interferon in the treatment of lymphomas, as with other neoplasms, tumor factors, host factors and treatment factors must be defined. Mechanisms of resistance and sensitivity to the antiproliferative action of interferon need to be further characterized in vitro. Similarly the role of the immune system and the potential for manipulation with interferon require further definition. For now, clinical studies must ensure that homogeneous patient populations are enrolled in carefully designed trials employing a variety of doses and schedules. Continued monitoring of antiproliferative and immunomodulatory effects in treated patients may provide retrospective insights. The clinical evaluation of the now plentiful and multiple interferons is a formidable task. Years of critical investigation will be required to obtain the ultimate answers.

REFERENCES

Blomgren, H., Cantell, K., Johannsen, B., Lagergren, C., Ringborg, U., and Strander, H. 1976, Interferon therapy in Hodgkin's disease, Acta. Med. Scand., 199:527.

Cantell, K., and Hirvonen, S. 1978, Large scale production of human leukocyte interferon containing 10 units per ml, J. Gen. Virol., 39:541.

Chirigos, M.A., and Pearson, J.W. 1973, Cure of murine leukemia with drug and interferon treatment, J. Natl. Cancer Inst., 51:1367.

Einhorn, S., and Strander, H. 1977, Is interferon tumor specific? Effect of human leukocyte and fibroblast interferon on the growth of lymphoblastoid and osteosarcoma cell lines, J. Gen. Virol., 35:573.

Einhorn, S., and Strander, H. 1978, Interferon therapy for neoplastic disease in man. In vitro and in vivo studies, Adv. Exp. Med. Biol., 110:159.

Gattiker, H.H., Wiltshaw, E., and Galton, D.A.G. 1980, Spontaneous regression in non-Hodgkin's lymphoma, Cancer, 45:2627.

Graff, S., Kanel, R., and Kastner, O. 1970, Interferon, Trans. NY Acad. Sci., 32:545.

Gresser, I., Coppey, J., and Bourali, C. 1969, Interferon and murine leukemia. VI. Effect of interferon preparations on the lymphoid leukemia of AKR mice, J. Natl. Cancer Inst., 43:1083.

Gresser, I., Chantal, M., and Tovey, M. 1978, Efficacy of combined interferon cyclophosphamide therapy after diagnosis of lymphoma in AKR mice, Eur. J. Cancer, 14:97.

Gutterman, J.U., Blumenschein, G.R., Alexanian, R., Yap, H., Buzdar, A.U., Cabanillas, F., Hortobagyi, G.N., Hersh, E.M., Rasmussen, S.L., Harmon, M., Kramer, M., and Pestka, S. 1980, Leukocyte interferon-induced tumor regression in human metastatic breast cancer, multiple myeloma and malignant lymphoma, Ann. Intern. Med., 93:399.

Gutterman, J.U., Fein, S., Quesada, J., Horning, S.J., Levine, J.F., Alexanian, R., Bernhardt, L., Kramer, M., Spiegel, H., Colburn, W., Trown, P., Merigan, T., and Dziewanowski, Z. 1982, Recombinant leukocyte A interferon: pharmacokinetics, single-dose tolerance, and biologic effects in cancer patients, Ann. Intern. Med., 96:549.

Horning, S.J., Levine, J.F., Miller, R.A., Rosenberg, S.A., and Merigan, T.C. 1982, Clinical and immunologic effects of recombinant leukocyte A interferon in eight patients with advanced cancer, JAMA, 247:1718.

Horoszewicz, J.S., Leong, S.S., and Carter, W.A. 1979, Noncycling tumor cells are sensitive targets for the antiproliferative activity of human interferon, Science, 206:1091.

Huddlestone, J.R., Merigan, T.C., and Oldstone, M.B.A. 1979, The induction and kinetics of natural killer cells in humans following interferon therapy, Nature, 282:417.

Krikorian, J.G., Portlock, C.S., Cooney, P., and Rosenberg, S.A. 1980, Spontaneous regression of non-Hodgkin's lymphoma: a report of nine cases, Cancer, 46:2093.

Louie, A.C., Gallagher, J.G., Sikora, K., Levy, R., Rosenberg, S.A., and Merigan, T.C. 1981, Follow-up observations on the effect on human leukocyte interferon in non-Hodgkin's lymphoma, Blood, 58:712.

Maluish, A., Conlon, J., Ortaldo, J.R., Sherwin, S.A., Leavitt, R., Fein, S., Weirnik, P., Oldham, R.K., and Herberman, R.B. 1982, Modulation of NK and monocyte activity in advanced cancer patients receiving interferon, in: "Interferons", p.377, T.C. Merigan, and R.M. Friedman, eds., Academic Press, New York.

Merigan, T.C., Sikora, K., Breeden, J.H., Levy, R., and Rosenberg, S.A. 1978, Preliminary observations on the effect of human leukocyte interferon in non-Hodgkin's lymphoma, N. Engl. J. Med., 299:1449.

Rasmussen, L.E., and Merigan, T.C. 1980, Effect of interferon therapy on circulating lymphocytes in humans, J. Interferon Res., 1:101.

Sherwin, S.A., Knost, J.A., Fein, S., Abrams, P.G., Foon, K.A., Ochs, J.J., Schoenberger, C., Maluish, A.E., and Oldham, R.K. 1982, A multiple-dose Phase I trial of recombinant luekocyte A interferon in cancer patients, JAMA, 248:2461.

Sikora, K., Basham, T., Dilley, J., Levy, R., and Merigan, T.C. 1980, Inhibition of lymphoma hybrids by human interferon, Lancet, 2:891.

LEUKEMIA

AMA ROHATINER

I.C.R.F. Department of Medical Oncology
St. Bartholomew's Hospital, London, EC1A

Much of the initial work on the anti-proliferative effects of
interferon (IFN) was carried out using mouse L1210 leukemia, a useful
model extensively for the study of anti-cancer agents (Waxman, 1975).
Some of these studies, together with those on virus-induced and
spontaneously occurring leukemias in mice will be reviewed. The in
vitro effects of IFN on human leukemia blast cells will then be
considered, prior to evaluating the preliminary results of clinical
trials in patients with lymphoid and myelogenous leukemia.

In a discussion of interferons and leukemia, it is perhaps
appropriate, first of all, to consider the effect of IFN on normal
haemopoietic tissue.

EFFECT OF INTERFERON ON THE NORMAL BONE MARROW

Myelosuppression has consistently been reported in clinical
trials with interferon, both in cancer patients (Priestman, 1980;
Gutterman et al., 1980; Horning et al., 1982) and in patients
receiving IFN as an anti-viral agent (Greenberg et al., 1976).
Neutropenia and thrombocytopenia have occasionally obliged treatment
to be stopped prematurely, and in patients receiving partially
purified IFN-α after allogeneic bone marrow transplantation,
restitution of bone marrow function was delayed (Nissen et al.,
1977). A number of studies have addressed the problem in vitro:-
Nissen et al. observed inhibition of granulocyte colony formation in
cultures of normal bone marrow when partially purified IFN-α was
added to the medium. The cytotoxic effects of IFN-α on granulocyte
progenitor cells have subsequently been confirmed (Greenberg et al.,
1977; van 't Hull et al., 1978; Verma et al., 1981; Oladipupo et al.,

1981). Comparison of the inhibitory effects of IFN's and β reveals conflicting results:- van 't Hull et al. (1978) found IFN-α to be more inhibitory than IFN-β for myeloid (CFU-C) progenitor cells, though the converse was recently reported (Oladipupo et al., 1981). Verma et al. (1981) observed wide variation in the sensitivity of CFU-C to both IFN's, and high doses of IFN-α and β were required to inhibit erythroid progenitor cells (CFU-E).

MURINE LEUKEMIA

Transplantable Tumors - In Vitro Studies

In the first of a series of studies with murine leukemia, Gresser demonstrated that mouse IFN inhibits multiplication of L1210 cells in culture (Gresser et al., 1970a). The degree of inhibition was found to correlate with the anti-viral titer of the IFN preparation, thus, a dose/response relationship for the degree of inhibition was established and was subsequently confirmed for human myeloblasts (Balkwill et al., 1977; Rohatiner et al., 1981).

Incubation of L1210 cells with IFN also resulted in a 100 fold decrease in their tumorigenicity and in their capacity to form colonies in semi-solid agar (Gresser et al., 1971).

Transplantable Tumors - In Vivo Studies

Daily intraperitoneal administration of IFN has been shown to inhibit the growth of several transplantable murine ascitic tumors including L1210 and to increase the survival of tumor-inoculated mice (Gresser et al., 1969; Gresser et al., 1970b). Interferon was only effective when continued after tumor inoculation. Optimal anti-tumor effects were achieved when contact between IFN and tumor cells was maximal (i.e. when both IFN and tumor were inoculated intra-peritoneally) although IFN also proved effective when administered at a site distant from that of implantation. IFN was most effective when the tumor mass was low. Under these conditions tumor-inoculated mice survived, whereas, once the tumor was well established, administration of IFN did not result in lysis or regression.

These results imply a direct anti-proliferative effect, but Gresser et al. have also reported an interesting experiment in which a transplantable L1210 leukemia that was IFN-resistant in vitro was still inhibited in vivo, although not to the same extent as a line that was IFN sensitive (Gresser et al., 1972). In the absence of a direct anti-proliferative effect, the anti-tumor effect was interpreted as having been mediated by enhancement of host immune function.

The growth inhibitory effect of IFN on mouse myeloid leukemic cells was demonstrated by Lotem and Sachs (1978), who stressed the differences in susceptibility between different clones of myeloid cells, even when these dervied from the same tumor. Differences in sensitivity to IFN have similarly been reported for myeloblasts derived from different individuals with acute myelogenous leukemia (AML) (Balkwill et al., 1977; Rohatiner et al., 1981).

Virus Induced Leukemias

Gresser and his co-workers also investigated the effect of IFN on the evolution of the Friend and Rauscher murine leukemias and the results may be summarized as follows:- repeated administration of IFN inhibited the development of splenomegaly in mice inoculated with Friend virus (Gresser et al., 1967). Even when IFN was initiated one week after viral inoculation, i.e. when splenomegaly had already developed, IFN still exerted a significant inhibitory effect.

Likewise, administration of IFN to mice infected with Rauscher virus prolonged mean survival time and delayed the development of hepatosplenomegaly, leukocytosis and anemia (Gresser et al., 1968).

Wheelock and Larke (1968) studied the effect of non-tumor viruses on virus-induced leukemia, postulating an IFN effect: mice with established Friend virus leukemia were inoculated with Sendai virus, resulting in prolongation of survival equivalent to that observed with IFN itself. This principle was also applied to a patient with refractory AML: sequential inoculation of six virus types was followed by transient clinical and haematological remission. However, although at autopsy the bone marrow showed no leukemic blast cells, the results are difficult to interpret because the patient also intermittently received 6-Mercaptopurine (Wheelock and Dingle, 1964).

Spontaneous Neoplasms

A 'protective' effect of IFN has also been reported for spontaneously occuring murine cancers in which a viral aetiology is implicated (Gresser et al., 1978a), including the leukemia of AKR mice which develop lymphoma/leukemia after the sixth month of life. Newborn AKR mice were treated with mouse IFN for three months:- the incidence of lymphoid leukemia was decreased and IFN significantly prolonged survival compared to that of untreated controls.

Perhaps of more relevance to the clinical situation is the observation that IFN treatment initiated after diagnosis of AKR lymphoma (i.e. thymic, enlargement, splenomegaly and lymphadenopathy) resulted in a 100% increase in survival time (Gresser et al., 1976). In mice with 'advanced leukemia' Graff et al. (1970) also observed rapid reduction in the size of nodes and the spleen in mice treated with greater than 10^5 units of IFN per day, together with a 14-fold prolongation of survival.

The problem with all such experiments involving leukemia of
viral aetiology is that the effect of IFN may have been mediated by
inhibition of viral replication and cellular transformation.
However, the anti-tumor effects described for transplantable tumors
(Gresser et al., 1970c; Gresser and Tovey, 1978b) suggest a direct
anti-proliferative effect on the tumor cells, though it is possible
that both mechanisms might be operating simultaneously.

Thus, IFN exerts anti-proliferative effects in experimental
animals injected with oncogenic viruses and transplantable tumor
cells, as well as in mice developing 'spontaneous', viral-associated
neoplastic disease. These results compare favorably with those
achieved using conventional chemotherapeutic agents. For example,
Frei et al. (1974) reported that four of 27 cytotoxic compounds
increased the mean survival of AKR mice after diagnosis of lymphoma
by 100% or more. Interferon had the same effect and could therefore
be considered a highly effective anti-tumor agent in this
experimental system. However, in animal studies, in virtually all
instances, complete regression of a well established tumor mass has
not been observed.

INTERFERON IN COMBINATION WITH CYTOTOXIC DRUGS

In murine models, IFN has been combined with conventional
cytotoxic agents. Chirigos and Pearson (1973) administered mouse IFN
after BCNU induced remission in a murine leukemia (LSTRA). Apparent
synergism was observed, with a significantly increased 'cure' rate
and doubling of survival time in mice receiving both treatment
modalities. Gresser et al. administered IFN and Cyclophosphamide to
mice with AKR lymphoma (Gresser et al., 1978b) - the survival time
was double that observed with either agent alone. The enhanced
therapeutic response achieved with IFN administered as adjuvant
therapy may theoretically have been due to an anti-proliferative
effect on residual malignant cells and/or to an IFN enhanced
macrophage and NK cell tumoricidal effect.

In order further to assess the interaction of IFN with
chemotherapeutic agents, mice with L1210 leukemia were treated with
Methotrexate (MTX), 6-Mercaptopurine (6MP), Adriamycin, Cytosine
Arabinoside, Cyclophosphamide, 6MP and MTX, or, each drug in
combination with mouse L-cell IFN (Slater et al., 1981). The
addition of IFN to all MTX containing regimens increased mean
survival time but IFN failed to enhance the response of L1210
leukemia to the other drugs tested.

IN VITRO EFFECTS OF INTERFERON ON HUMAN LEUKEMIC BLAST CALLS

In 1977, Balkwill and Oliver demonstrated an *in vitro* cytostatic
effect on myeloblasts using IFN derived from a Namalwa lymphoblastoid

cell line, Hu IFN-α N. Later, in the context of a Phase I study of
Hu IFN-α N in patients with haematological malignancies the following
observations were made (Rohatiner et al., 1981). In patients with
AML, bone marrow and peripheral blood myeloblasts were cultured with
Hu IFN-α N at concentrations of 10, 10^2, 10^3 and 10^4 units/ml.
Growth was assessed by uptake of tritiated thymidine and viable cell
counts at three days. Interferon decreased cell survival and
inhibited thymidine uptake at concentrations greater than 10
units/ml. Growth inhibition was dose dependent, 50% inhibition
occurring at an in vitro concentration of 10^3 units/ml, a level that
can be achieved in the serum of patients receiving Hu IFN-α N when
doses of greater than 30 x 10^6 units/m^2/day are administered by
continuous intravenous infusion (Rohatiner et al., 1982).

A comparative study of the effects of IFNs α and β on short-term
cultures of leukemic blasts (AML) showed a marked difference in
sensitivity between individuals and IFN-β appeared to be a more
effective suppressor of DNA synthesis (Lundgren et al., 1980).

Both normal and leukemic (CML) human clonogenic cells exhibit a
decrease in granulocyte colony forming capacity when exposed to IFN's
α and β (Greenberg et al., 1977; Oladipupo et al., 1981) IFN-β has
also been shown to inhibit both primary proliferation and self-
renewal of blast progenitors in a colony forming assay of myelogenous
blast cells (Taetle et al., 1980).

Recently, Lee et al. (1982) using natural buffy coat IFN-α and
purified IFN-α subtypes have shown differential inhibitory effects on
a B cell lymphoblastoid cell line and cell lines derived from B and T
cell acute lymphoblastic leukemias.

Thus, in vitro, interferon appears to be an effective anti-
proliferative agent.

CLINICAL TRIALS IN PATIENTS WITH LEUKEMIA

CLL:- Following reports of responses to IFN-α in small numbers
of patients with other B cell malignancies (Mellstedt et al., 1979;
Louie et al., 1981), Gutterman et al. (1980) reported transient
responses, i.e. a fall in the circulating lymphocyte count (both
patients) and a reduction in the size of enlarged lymph nodes (one
patient) in two out of four patients treated with IFN-α. A study of
recombinant DNA leukocyte IFN (IFN-α 2) in patients with CLL has
recently commenced at St. Bartholomew's Hospital, London.

CML:- A study of IFN-α 2 is currently in progress at St.
Bartholomew's Hospital. Patients with CML in chronic phase receive
100 x 10^6 U/m^2/day by continuous intravenous infusion for seven days.
A rapid fall in the white cell count has been observed but the

responses have been short lived, the white cell count returning to pre-treatment values within one to 12 weeks. To date there has been no change in the degree of splenomegaly or in the appearance of the bone marrow.

A study in progress at M.D. Anderson Hospital (Talpaz et al., 1982) using IFN-α 2 has also demonstrated an anti-proliferative effect in CML. Responding patients have been "maintained" on thrice weekly IFN-α 2 at doses between 3 and 9 x 10^6 units. As with conventional agents it appears to be possible to control the level of the white cell count. The long term results are awaited with interest.

ALL:- Hill et al. (1978) using partially purified IFN-α at a daily dose of 1 x 10^6 U/kg treated two children with ALL and observed a response in one patient. A further five patients were subsequently reported to have responded to IFN administered at half the dose (Hill et al., 1981). Whether the responses constituted complete remission or only a fall in the circulating blast cell count was not specified.

Five patients with ALL took part in the Phase I study of Hu IFN-α N (Rohatiner et al., 1982). A significant fall in the number of circulating leukemic blasts was observed in two patients who received daily doses of 15 and 200 x 10^6 U/m respectively for five days. However, there was no change in the degree of bone marrow infiltration but one cannot draw meaningful conclusions on the basis of such small numbers of patients.

AML:- With a view to possibly incorporating Hu IFN-α N into the management of patients with AML, a Phase I study was commenced at St. Bartholomew's Hospital in November 1980. Continuous intravenous infusion was selected as the schedule of choice because of the practical problem of thrombocytopenia in patients with acute leukemia and the theoretical advantage of prolonged exposure of the blast cells to IFN. The objectives of the study were to determine the maximum safely tolerated dose, toxicity and pharmacokinetics of intravenous Hu IFN-α N. In addition bone marrow and where possible, peripheral blood myeloblasts where cultured with Hu IFN-α N (as described above) prior to the patients' receiving interferon. The results may be summarized as follows:

A maximum tolerated dose of 100 x 10^6 units/m^2/day, administered by continuous intravenous infusion for seven days was established.

Peak serum interferon levels of 10^3 U/ml were achieved in the majority of patients who received daily doses greater than 30 x 10^6 U/m^2.

In vitro, interferon exerted a growth inhibitory effect in all 21 patients tested at concentrations greater than 10 U/ml. Although there was variation in sensitivity between patients, approximately 50% inhibition was observed at concentrations of 10^3 U/ml.

Although this was principally a Phase I study, a comment on response is perhaps justified:- The majority of patients showed no response. Of six evaluable patients with AML who received between 50 and 200 x 10^6 U/m^2/day for seven to ten days, three patients showed no response. In two patients there was a considerable fall in the circulating blast cell count but no change in the degree of bone marrow infiltration. In one patient (who received 50 x 10^6 U/m^2/day for ten days) clearing of blasts from the peripheral blood was associated with a decrease in the degree of bone marrow infiltration from 99% blasts (hypercellular) to less than 5% blasts (normoceullar). A mass on the anterior chest wall decreased in size during the interferon infusion but never regressed completely. The patient was therefore not in complete remission. Three weeks later a further infusion at a dose of 100 x 10^6 U/m^2 was administered for five days but peripheral blood and bone marrow relapse occurred at three months. A Phase II study is currently in progress in patients with AML who have either failed to enter remission with conventional therapy or who have relapsed following such therapy.

In conclusion, it is still too early to know whether interferon will have any place in the treatment of patients with leukemia. Certainly some biological activity has been demonstrated in very small numbers of patients and these preliminary results warrant further investigation in careful clinical trials. When these are reported, however, it should perhaps be remembered that a demonstration of "biological activity" does not necessarily imply a meaningful response.

ACKNOWLEDGEMENT

I am very grateful to Jane for typing the manuscript, again and again.

REFERENCES

Balkwill, F., and Oliver, R.T.O. 1977, Interferons as cell regulatory molecules, Int. J. Cancer, 20:500.
Chirigos, M.A., and Pearson, J.W. 1973, Cure of murine leukemia with drug and interferon treatment, J. Natl. Cancer Inst., 51:1367.
Frei, E., III, Schabel, F.M. Jr., and Goldin, A. 1974, Comparative chemotherapy of AKR lymphoma and human hematological neoplasia, Cancer Res., 34:184.
Graff, S., Kassel, R., and Kastner, O. 1970, Interferon, Trans. N.Y. Acad. Sci., [2], 32:545.

Greenberg, H.B., Pollard, R.B., Lutwick, L.I., Gregory, P.B.,
    Robinson, W.S., and Merigan, T.C. 1976, Effect of human
    leukocyte interferon on hepatitis B virus infection in patients
    with chronic active hepatitis, N. Engl. J. Med., 295:517.
Greenberg, P.L., and Mosny, S.A. 1977, Cytotoxic effects of
    interferon in vitro on granulocytic progenitor cells, Cancer
    Res., 37:1794.
Gresser, I., Falcoff, R., Fontaine-Brouty-Boye, D., Zajdela, F.,
    Coppey, J., and Falcoff, E. 1967, Interferon and murine leukemia
    IV. Further studies on the efficacy of interferon preparations
    administered after inoculation of Friend virus, Proc. Soc. Exp.
    Biol. Med., 126:791.
Gresser, I., Berman, I., De The, G., Brouty-Boye, D., Coppey, J., and
    Falcoff, E. 1968, Interferon and murine leukemia V. Effect of
    interferon preparations on the evolution of Raushcer Disease in
    mice, J. Natl. Cancer Inst., 41:505.
Gresser, I., Bourali, C., Levy, J.P., Brouty-Boye, D., and Thomas,
    M-T. 1969, Increased survival in mice inoculated with tumor
    cells and treated with interferon preparation, Proc. Natl. Acad.
    Sci. USA, 63:51.
Gresser, I., Brouty-Boye, D., Thomas, M-T., and Macierira-Coelho, A.
    1970a, Interferon and cell division, I. Inhibition of the
    multiplication of mouse leukemia L1210 cells in vitro by
    interferon preparations, Proc. Natl. Acad. Sci. USA, 66:1052.
Gresser, I., Bourali, C., Chouroulinkov, I., Brouty-Boye, D., and
    Thomas, M-T. 1970b, Treatment of neoplasia in mice with an
    interferon preparation, Ann. N.Y. Acad. Sci., 173:694.
Gresser, I., and Bourali, C. 1970c, Antitumour effects of interferon
    preparations in mice, J. Natl. Cancer Inst., 45:365.
Gresser, I., Thomas, M-T., and Brouty-Boye, D. 1971, Effect of
    interferon treatment of L1210 cells in vitro on tumor and colony
    formation, Nature (New Biol.), 231:20.
Gresser, I., Maury, C., and Brouty-Boye, D. 1972, Mechanism of the
    antitumour effect of interferon in mice, Nature, 239:167.
Gresser, I., Maury, C., and Towey, M.G. 1976, Interferon and murine
    leukemia VII. Therapeutic effect of interferon preparations
    after diagnosis of lymphoma in AKR mice, Int. J. Cancer, 17:647.
Gresser, I., and Tovey, M.G., 1978a, Antitumour effects of
    interferon, Biochem. Biophys. Acta., 516:231.
Gresser, I., Maury, C., and Tovey, M. 1978b, Efficacy of combined
    interferon cyclophosphamide therapy after diagnosis of lymphoma
    in AKR mice, Eur. J. Cancer, 14:97.
Gutterman, J.U., Blumenschein, G.R., Alexanian, R., Yap, Y.P.,
    Buzdar, A.U., Cabanillas, F., Hortoagyi, G.M., Hersh, E.M.,
    Rasmussen, S.L., Harmon, M., Kramer, M., and Pestka, S. 1980,
    Leucocyte interferon-induced tumor regression in human
    metastatic breast cancer, multiple myeloma and malignant
    lymphoma, Ann. Intern. Med., 93:388.
Hill, N.O., Loeb, E., Pardue, A., Khan, A., Dorn, G.L., Comparini,
    S., and Hill, J.M. 1978, Leukocyte interferon production and its
    effectiveness in acute lymphatic leukemia, J. Clin. Hematol.
    Oncol., 8:67.

Hill, N.O., Pardue, A., Khan, A., Aleman, D., and Hill, J.M. 1981, High-dose human leukocyte interferon trials in leukemia and cancer, Med. Pediatr. Oncol., 9:1.

Horning, S.J., Levine, J.F., Miller, R.A., and Merigan, T. 1982, Clinical and immunological effects of recombinant leucocyte interferon in eight patients with advanced cancer, J.A.M.A., 42:1312.

Lee, S.H., Kelley, S., Chiu, H., and Stebbing, N. 1982, Stimulation of natural cell killer activity and inhibition of proliferation of various leukaemic cells by purified human leukocyte interferon subtypes, Cancer Research, 42:1312.

Lotem, J., and Sachs, L. 1978, Genetic dissociation of different cellular effects of interferon on myeloid leukaemic cells, Int. J. Cancer, 22:214.

Louie, A.C., Gallagher, J.G., Sikora, K., Levy, R., Rosenberg, S.A., and Merigan, T.C. 1981, Follow up observations on the effect of human leukocyte interferon in non-Hodgkin's lymphoma, Blood, 58:712.

Lundgren, E., Hillorn, W., Holmberg, D., Lenner, P., and Roos, G. 1980, Comparative study on the effects of fibroblast and leukocyte interferon on short term cultures of leukaemic cells, Ann. N.Y. Acad. Sci., 350, 628.

Mellstedt, H., Bjorkholm, M., Johansson, E., Ahre, A., Holm, G., and Strander, H. 1979, Interferon therapy in myelomatosis, Lancet, 1:245.

Nissen, C., Speck, B., Emodi, G., and Iscove, N.N. 1977, Toxicity of human leucocyte interferon preparations in human bone marrow cultures, Lancet, 1977:203.

Oladipupo, W.C.K., Svet-Moldavskaya, I., Vilcek, J., Ohnuma Takao and Holland, J.F. 1981, Inhibitory effects of human leukocyte and fibroblast interferons on normal and chronic myelogenous leukaemic granulocytic progenitor cells, Oncology, 38:356.

Priestman, T.J. 1980, Initial evaluation of human lymphoblastoid interferon in patients with advanced malignant disease, Lancet, II:113.

Rohatiner, A.Z.S., Balkwill, F.R., Malpas, J.S., and Lister, T.A. 1981, in: "Modern Trends in Human Leukemia, Vol. IV", Springer, Heidelberg.

Rohatiner, A.Z.S., Balkwill, F.R., Griffin, D.D., Malpas, J.S., and Lister, T.A. 1982, A Phase I study of human lymphoblastoid interferon administered by continuous intravenous infusion, Cancer Chenother. Pharmacol., 9:97.

Slater, L.M., Wetzel, M.W., and Cesario, T. 1981, Combined interferon - antimetabolite therapy of murine L1210 leukemia, Cancer, 48:5.

Taetle, R., Buick, R.N., and McCullock, E.A. 1980, Effect of interferon on colony formation in culture by blast cell progenitors in acute myeloblastic leukemia, Blood, 56:549.

Talpaz, M., McCredie, K.B., and Gutterman, J.U. 1982, Clinical investigation of human leucocyte interferon in chronic myelogenous leukemia. (Abstract) Data presented at the 3rd International Congress for Interferon Research No. 1982.

van't Hull, E., Schelleckens, H., Lowenberg, B., and de Vries, M.J.
    1978, Influence of interferon preparations on the proliferative
    capacity of human and mouse bone marrow cells in vitro, Cancer
    Research, 38:911.
Verma, D.S., Spitzer, G., and Gutterman, J.U. 1981, Measurement of
    effect of human leukocyte interferon on human granulocyte
    colony-forming cells in vitro, in: "Methods in enzymology, 79,
    pt 3, 520.
Waxman, S. 1975, in: "Clinical Cancer Chemotherapy", p.17, E.M.
    Greenspan, ed., Raven Press, New York.
Wheelock, E.F., and Larke, R.P. 1968, Efficacy of interferon in the
    treatment of mice with established Friend virus leukemia, Proc.
    Soc. Exp. Biol. Med., 127:230.
Wheelock, E.F., and Dingle, J.H. 1964, Observations on the repeated
    administration of viruses to a patient with acute leukemia,
    N.E.J. Med., 271:645.

MYELOMA

TERENCE J. PRIESTMAN

Department of Radiotherapy and Oncology, Queen Elizabeth
and Dudley Road Hospitals, Birmingham

CLINICAL BACKGROUND

Multiple myeloma is one of a group of disorders known
collectively as plasma-cell dyscrasias. These conditions range from
the highly malignant to the completely benign but all are
characterized by unbalanced proliferation of those B-lymphocytes
which produce gamma-globulin (immunoglobulin). The excess of plasma
cells leads to increase production of various immunoglobulins or
homologous peptide subunits of these proteins. This over production
is usually associated with a deficiency of normal immunoglobulin.
Multiple myeloma may be diagnosed when two of the following three
criteria are present:-

(a) The presence of abnormal plasma-cells, or excessive numbers
of normal plasma cells in the bone marrow.

(b) A monoclonal immunoglobulin in the serum, the urine, or
both.

(c) Radiological evidence of osteolytic lesions unexplained by
other causes.

The classification of individual subtypes of myeloma is based upon
analysis of immunoglobulin levels. 80 per cent of patients have
abnormally elevated levels of immunoglobulin (Ig) in the blood, the
majority of these exhibit high levels of IgG (65% of patients) with
excess of IgA as the next commonest finding (33%); raised IgD and IgE
levels are rare. In addition 50% of patients will have Bence-Jones
protein (a peptide subunit of immunoglobulin) in their urine and in a
proportion of cases this is the only protein abnormality.

Multiple myeloma is multicentric from its outset and although usually initially confined to bone, over 60 per cent of patients will develop extraskeletal involvement (most commonly in the spleen, lymph nodes, kidney and lungs). The disease is uniformly fatal, although in patients without renal involvement, cytotoxic chemotherapy has increased median survival times to three – four years compared to less than 12 months when local radiotherapy and supportive care were the only measures available.

A number of factors make assessment of new therapy for myeloma particularly difficult. These include:-

(a) The relative rarity of the tumor: in England and Wales its incidence is only 3.4 per 100,000.

(b) The lack of a universally agreed staging system for the disease: although features such as renal impairment, anemia and low serum albumin levels are all recognized as adverse prognostic factors there is no uniform system for defining the extent of disease prior to therapy although various methods have proposed ranging from a simple grading based on the presence or absence of renal failure to computer programmes designed to assess the actual plasma cell mass (Salmon and Wampler, 1977).

(c) The lack of universally agreed criteria of response: the diffuse nature of the disease and the multiplicity of its direct and indirect manifestations have made the definition of precise response criteria difficult. Most authors have concentrated on direct effects and based their assessment on falls in serum or urine myeloma protein, reduction in the proportion of plasma cells in the bone marrow and radiological evidence of bone healing but the number of parameters needed to show improvement and the degree of change required before a benefit may be claimed have varied in different series. In addition some groups have insisted on improvement in indirect manifestations, such as anemia, weight loss and abnormal blood calcium levels, before recording a response.

In the several series evaluating interferons the criteria of response, stages of disease and extent of previous therapy have all differed. In addition the type of interferon used and even the potency and purity of individual preparations have varied. All these differences must be taken into account when considering the results so far reported and in order to gain an accurate impression of what has been achieved it is necessary to consider each study individually.

INITIAL REPORTS OF INTERFERON ACTIVITY IN MYELOMA

During 1979 and 1980 three groups published encouraging results using leukocyte interferon in patients with myeloma. In each of

these studies the interferon used was supplied by the Finnish Red
Cross Blood Transfusion Service and contained a mixture of alpha-
interferons with specific activities ranging from 2.5 x 10^5 to 1 x
10^6 IU/mg protein (approximately 1% pure interferon). The
preparation was given by intramuscular injection at doses ranging
from 3 - 6 x 10^6 units daily.

Mellstedt et al. reported on four cases and saw complete
remissions in two patients and partial remissions in the others. In
one patient with IgA disease there was complete disappearance of
myeloma protein from the blood and a fall in bone marrow plasma cells
from 40% to zero, the remission having been sustained for nine months
at the time of reporting. In a patient with Bence-Jones myeloma
abnormal protein was cleared from the urine, plasma cells fell from
30% to 2% in the marrow and the response lasted over a year. The
partial responses were seen in patients with IgG and IgA myeloma and
had lasted 15 and 19 months respectively (Mellstedt et al., 1979).
All these patients received interferon as first line therapy. In the
initial report of the study sponsored by the American Cancer Society
nine out of 11 patients had also received no prior chemotherapy. In
this series disease regression was noted in three patients and
stabilisation of progressive disease recorded in two others but no
further details were given (Osserman et al., 1980). An M.D. Anderson
Hospital series gave the results of treatment on ten patients but in
this study only three patients received interferon as initial
therapy, of the remainder three had proved unresponsive to the
combination of alkylating agents and steroids and four had relapsed
after initially successful cytotoxic therapy. Three responses were
seen with greater than 50% reductions in myeloma protein in two
patients with IgG disease and one with Bence-Jones myeloma. The
remission durations were 24 and 63+ weeks for the IgG patients and
52+ weeks for the patient with Bence-Jones proteinurea. Interestingly the latter was the only one of the responders who had not
received previous therapy, one of the IgG patients had been resistant
to cytotoxics and the other had relapsed (Gutterman et al., 1980).

Appearing within a few months of one another these three
publications clearly demonstrated that leukocyte interferon had
activity in multiple myeloma and the further results from these
groups were eagerly awaited in order to clarify the extent of that
activity. Two of the centers have now reported additional data.

UPDATED RESULTS

The Scandinavians extended their initial pilot study from four
to 13 patients and included in this group five patients who had
relapsed after previous cytotoxic therapy. Of the previously
untreated patients five out of eight showed a response (although this
group included the four patients reported initially) whereas in the

relapsing patients only one showed an objective benefit. These results were considered sufficiently encouraging to justify a prospectively randomized trial comparing interferon with melphalan and prednisolone as first-line therapy. The initial results of this study reported on 43 evaluable patients. In the melphalan-prednisolone group six out of 21 had responded, compared to four out of 22 in the interferon arm. There is no information on the duration of response but in the interferon group 15 patients had died at the time of reporting compared to only nine in the cytotoxic group although statistical analysis showed no significant difference in the overall survival times (p = 0.1). The initial prognostic variables were comparable for the two sets of patients (Mellstedt et al., 1982).

The MD Anderson study was prolonged to include a total of 21 patients (Alexanian et al., 1982). Twelve were previously untreated, five had relapsed after an initial response to melphalan and prednisone and four had proved unresponsive to this regime. Of the previously untreated patients three showed objective regression of disease and one patient in each of the other two groups had a greater than 50 per cent reduction in myeloma protein. Of the eight previously untreated patients who were resistant to interferon four subsequently gained good partial responses with cytotoxic therapy. The duration of interferon-induced remissions lasted from three to 33 months, during which time the patients were maintained on a dose of 3 mega units three times each week.

These figures show a decline in response rates from 100% to 18% in the Swedish series and from 30% to 24% in the Texas study. This may well simply represent the emergence of a more accurate view of the level of interferon activity with increasing numbers of patients and that an expectation of a 20 - 25% response rate is probably realistic. One complicating factor, however, relates to the formulation of the interferon used in the Swedish randomized study and the latter part of the M.D. Anderson series. In both instances a change was made from wet-filled to lyophilized material and subsequent analysis has shown that in some batches the freeze-drying process led to a greater than 50 per cent loss of interferon activity in the preparation (Alexanian, 1982). Whether better results would have been achieved had the liquid material been used throughout must remain speculative.

OTHER INTERFERONS IN MYELOMA

A number of papers have included patients with myeloma in miscellaneous series and on occasions responses have been claimed but such anecdotal results are difficult to interpret and will not be reviewed here. Three papers have evaluated β interferons in myeloma. In two series no responses were seen in ten (Billiau et al., 1981)

and five (Ezaki et al., 1982) patients respectively. In the third
group four out of 16 patients showed a greater than 50% reduction in
bone marrow plasmacytosis but in no instance was there a corresponding fall in myeloma protein levels (Misset et al., 1981). There
seems little prospect that β interferon has a role to play in
multiple myeloma.

The evaluation of recombinant interferons is still at an early
stage and most reports are confined to a discussion of their
pharmacology and toxicity. One recent study has, however, given
details of the therapeutic response using the Hoffmann La Roche/
Genentech recombinant preparation IFLrA. Although seven of 16
patients with several tumor types showed objective evidence of tumor
regression during the study none of the four patients with myeloma
who were included in this series responded (Gutterman et al., 1982).

Human lymphoblastoid interferon is at present being evaluated in
a Phase II study in myeloma in the United Kingdom. So far five
patients have been entered but no responses have been seen. The
study is, however, restricted to those patients who have failed to
respond to or relapsed after, conventional cytotoxic and steroid
therapy (Priestman, 1982).

SUMMARY AND PROSPECTS

The initial extremely good results from interferon administration in multiple myeloma have not been sustained but even so it
is still likely that an overall response rate of 20 to 25 per cent is
possible. The fact that responses have been seen in a number of
patients with disease resistant to, or relapsed after, conventional
therapy increases the likelihood that myeloma is one condition where
interferons may find a useful therapeutic role.

Whether the present results may be enhanced by changes in
interferon preparations or other approaches remains speculative but
certainly a number of possibilities have still to be explored.
Evaluation of recombinant interferons is at an early stage; recent
studies have shown that very high doses of lymphoblastoid interferon
may be given by intravenous infusion (Rohatiner et al., 1982) the
therapeutic potential of discovery may be considerable; methods are
being devised for in vitro testing of individual patients myeloma
cells to detect those sensitive to interferons allowing greater
selectivity in treatment (Durie et al., 1982) and the potential for
combining interferons and cytotoxics which has looked so promising in
the laboratory has hardly been explored in the clinic. Whether
further study of these aspects will enhance present results is still
uncertain but already the clinical studies with leukocyte interferons
strongly suggest that they may have a part to play in the overall
management of myelomatosis.

REFERENCES

Alexanian, R., Gutterman, J., and Levy, H. 1982, Interferon treatment
    for multiple myeloma, Clinics in Haematology, II:211.
Billiau, A., Bloemmen, J., Bogaerts, M., Claeys, H., Van Damme, J.,
    De Ley, M., de Somer, P., Drochmans, A., Heremans, H., Kriel,
    A., Schetz, J., Tricot, G., Vermylen, C., Verwilghen, R., and
    Waer, M. 1981, Interferon therapy in multiple myeloma: Failure
    of human fibroblast interferon administration to alter the
    course of light chain disease, Eur. J. Cancer, 17:875.
Durie, B., Vaught, L., Soehnlen B, and Salmon S. 1982, Sensitivity to
    interferons and bisantrene in refractory myeloma: comparison
    between thymidine suppression, myeloma stem cell culture and
    clinical results, Proceedings American Association for Cancer
    Research, 23:116.
Ezaki, K., Ogawa, M., Okabe, K., Abe, K., Inove, K., Horikoshi, N.,
    and Inagaki, J. 1982, Clinical and immunological studies of
    human fibroblast interferon, Cancer Chemotherapy and
    Pharmacology, 8:47.
Gutterman, J., Blumenschein, G., Alexanian, R., Yap, H., Buzdar, A.,
    Cababillas, F., Hortobagyi, G., Hersh, E., Rasmussen, S.,
    Harman, M., Karmer, M., and Pestka, S. 1980, Leukocyte
    interferon-induced tumor regression in human metastatic breast
    cancer, multiple myeloma and malignant lymphoma, Annals of
    Internal Medicine, 93:399.
Gutterman, J., Fine, S., Quesada, J., Horning, S., Levine, J.,
    Alexanian, R., Bernhardt, L., Kramer, M., Spiegel, H., Colburn,
    W., Trown, P., Merigan, T., and Dziewanowska, Z. 1982,
    Recombinant leukocyte A interferon: pharmacokinetics,
    single-dose tolerance and biologic effects in cancer patients,
    Annals of Internal Medicine, 96:549.
Mellstedt, H., Bjorkholm, M., Johansson, B., Ahre, A., Holm, G., and
    Strander, H. 1979, Interferon therapy in myelomatosis, Lancet,
    1:245.
Mellstedt, H., Ahre, A., Bjorkholm, M., Johansson, B., Strander, H.,
    Brenning, G., Engstedt, L., Gahrton, G., Holm, G., Lehrner, R.,
    Longvist, B., Nordenskjold, B., Killander, A., Stalfeldt, A-M.,
    Simonsson, B., Ternstedt, B., and Wadman, B. 1982, Interferon
    therapy of patients with myeloma in Terry, W. and Rosenberg, S.
    Eds. Immunotherapy of human cancer, Elsevier North Holland
    Inc., New York, 387.
Misset, J., Gastriaburu, J., De Vassal, F., Mathe, G. 1981, Phase II
    trial of interferon (IF) in malignant gammopathics meningeal
    leukemia on chronic lymphatic leukemia (CLL), Proceedings
    American Association for Cancer Research, 22:491.
Osserman, E., Sherman, W., Alexanian, R., Gutterman, J., and Humphry,
    R. 1980, Preliminary results of the American Cancer Society
    (ACS) - sponsored trial of human leukocyte interferon (IF) in
    multiple myeloma (MM), Proceedings American Association for
    Cancer Research, 21:161.

Priestman, T. 1982, The present status of clinical studies with
    interferons in cancer in Britain, Philosophical Transactions of
    the Royal Society of London, Series B, 299:119.
Rohatiner, A., Balkwill, F., Griffin, D., Malpass, J., and Lister,
    T., 1982, A phase I study of human lymphoblastoid interferon
    administered by continuous intravenous infusion, Cancer
    Chemotherapy and Pharmacology, in press.
Salmon, S. and Wampler, S. 1977, Multiple myeloma: quantitive
    staging and assessment of response with a programmable pocket
    calculator, Blood, 49:379.

ERNEST C. BORDEN, JORDAN U. GUTTERMAN, JAMES F. HOLLAND
AND THOMAS L. DAO

University of Wisconsin Clinical Cancer Center, Madison
M.D. Anderson Hospitals and Tumor Institute, Houston
Mount Sinai Hospital and School of Medicine, New York
and Roswell Park Memorial Institute, Buffalo

The American Cancer Society began a review in 1978 of all data
regarding the antimitotic effect of interferons, the effect of
interferons on immuno-effector cells, the activity of interferons
against animal tumors, and the results of preliminary clinical trials
of interferons in the United States and Europe. At the conclusion of
this review, a decision was made to initiate an interferon clinical
trials program. Four tumor types were chosen for the initial
clinical study: lymphomas, myeloma, melanoma and breast carcinoma.

Several observations suggested that interferons might have antitumor activity agaomst breast carcinoma (Borden et al., 1981).
Female mice of the R III strain, which have a high spontaneous
incidence of mammary carcinoma, had a significant delay in
development of tumors when treated weekly from six weeks of age with
mouse interferon (Came and Moore, 1972). Although all treated mice
eventually developed carcinoma, median time to tumor appearance was
inhibited approximately six weeks (Table I). Athymic nude mice
receiving human breast carcinoma xenografts, were treated daily with
2×10^4 units of human interferon α (lymphoblastoid) (Balkwill et
al., 1980). Tumor development in treated mice was delayed and
inhibited (Table I). Of three different human tumors, two were
sensitive to interferon. In the sensitive tumors, the number of
tumors and weights of tumor were markedly decreased. Consistent with
this apparently direct antiproliferative effect of interferons in the
nude mouse was the inhibition of human breast carcinoma cell lines in
vitro (Balkwill et al., 1978). All three of the human breast
carcinoma cell lines tested were inhibited in growth by interferon α
(lymphoblastoid). Two of the carcinoma cell lines were inhibited in

103

TABLE I

Interferons in Experimental Breast Carcinoma Models

Breast Carcinoma Models	IFN	Result	Reference
Spontaneous RIII mouse	10^4 units weekly	Delay in tumor appearance	Came & Moore
Human tumors in nude mouse	2×10^4 units daily	Decreased tumor size and number	Balkwill et al
Human cells in vitro	100 units/ml	50% decrease in cell no. in 3 malignant lines at 7d	Balkwill et al

growth approximately 50% by 100 units of interferon α. Growth of
normal breast fibroblasts and epithelium were inhibited to about the
same extent as the malignant cells.

Two independent trials were begun, initially at M.D. Anderson
Hospital (Gutterman et al., 1980) and subsequently by the American
Cancer Society (Borden et al., 1982). The primary objective of these
trials was to confirm or refute the effectiveness of interferon α as
single agent therapy in inducing regressions in breast carcinoma.
Secondary objectives were to determine toxicities and pharmacokinetics of interferon α and to correlate disease response with
toxicities, pharmacokinetics, and immunologic effects of interferon
α. This review will present a combined analysis of these two trials.

At the time these trials were initiated, interferon α, prepared
from buffy coats, was the only interferon available with demonstrated
antitumor activity in man. It was obtained from the Finnish National
Red Cross (Cantell et al., 1973). It had been partially purified to
a specific activity of 10^6 units/mg of protein. Frozen and
lyophilized aliquots were packaged three million units per vial and
were safety tested both in Finland and in the United States. Batch
and viral testing confirmed absence of microbial contamination,
animal toxicity, unacceptable pyrogenicity after intravenous
injection of rabbits and limulus test, and hepatitis-B virus antigen
titers by complement fixation. Limited supplies of buffy coat
interferons prevented Phase I studies of optimal dose, route, and
schedule. Trials in osteosarcoma (Strander et al., 1978) had
administered interferons by daily intramuscular injection during the
induction phase. Intramuscular injection resulted in interferon
levels which reached their peak titer at three to six hours after
administration. Therefore this route and schedule were chosen for
initial trials.

Activity of a new therapy for oncologic patients with metastatic disease is determined by unrandomized evaluation of the drug in patients with histologically confirmed, objectively quantifiable disease. Patients eligible for the trial were those with recurrent disease quantifiable by measurement of soft tissue, lymph node, or pulmonary masses. The design for the American Cancer Society trial consisted of three million units of leukocyte interferon given intramuscularly daily. The initial duration of treatment was 28 days. At the end of this time, interferon was discontinued in any patient with progressive disease. Patients with stable disease or positive response were continued on interferon. If at the end of 42 days a patient still had stable disease, interferon was discontinued. All patients with partial response after the initial 42-day period were continued on interferon for a time equal to that required to achieve the partial response. The maximum that any patient could receive interferon was therefore 84 days for the American Cancer Society trial. The earlier M.D. Anderson trial had utilized either three or nine million units of interferon for induction for four - 12 weeks. In contrast to the American Cancer Society trial, a maintenance dose of 3 x 10 units interferon was continued three times a week in responders.

Twenty-six patients were entered in the American Cancer Society trial. Three were not considered in the final evaluation. One had received cytotoxic chemotherapy for metastatic disease and was thus

TABLE II

Phase II Evaluation of Human Leukocyte
Interferon in Metastatic Breast Carcinoma

Characteristics of Patients
(n = 40)

Age (yrs)			Menopause		Estrogen Receptor Status		Disease-free interval (mos)		
Range	Mean	Median	Yes	No	Pos	Neg	Range	Mean	Median
31-75	56	56	36	4	12	8	0-96	32	26

Prior Treatment			Dominant Metastatic Sites	
Mx	XRT	Cx	Soft Tissue	Visceral
36	21	6	21	19

not eligible for this trial. One did not have measurable disease, and the X-rays of one could not be located for review (clinically these patients, respectively progressed, improved, and had an objective partial response). The M.D. Anderson trial included 17 patients. A combined analysis could thus be undertaken of 23 plus 17 patients or a total of 40 (Table II). The age of the 40 entered patients ranged from 31 to 75 years with a median of 56 years. Most were postmenopausal and when estrogen receptor status was determined, 12 patients were positive and eight were negative. The mean disease-free interval was 31 months, with a median of 26 months. Dominant metastatic disease was in soft tissue sites in 21 patients and visceral sites in 19 patients.

Using the definitions of response codified by the International Union Against Cancer and the Breast Cancer Task Force of the United States, there were 11 objective partial responses (50% or greater reduction in the product of the diameter of the measurable tumor) in the two trials (Table III). Five additional patients had evidence of antitumor effect but not enough to qualify as an objective partial response. Responses were noted at both visceral and soft tissue sites including lymph nodes, chest wall, pleura, biopsy-confirmed bladder involvement, primary breast involvement and pulmonary involvement. The median duration of response in the American Cancer Society trial of interferon was 91 days with a range of 14 - 176 days. In the M.D. Anderson trial, where a maintenance period of interferon was given, the median duration of response was 196 days, with a range of 56 days to 756 days (Table IV).

TABLE III

Phase II Evaluation of Human Leukocyte Interferon
in Metastatic Breast Carcinoma

	Objective Disease Status on Interferon			
Trial	Total	Partial Response	Improvement	Stable or Progression
ACS	23	5	4	14
MDA	17	6	1	10
	40	11	5	24

No correlation of response or progression to estrogen receptor status, disease free interval, or dose escalation to 9×10^6 units.

TABLE IV

Phase II Evaluation of Human Leukocyte Interferon
in Metastatic Breast Carcinoma*

Response Duration					
Duration (days)		Duration off IFN (days)		MDA Trial - Maintenance 3 x/week** Duration (days)	
Median	Range	Median	Range	Median	Range
58	14-176	58	14-148	196	56-756

* n = 40; 3-9 x 10^6 units;   ** 3 x 10^6 units

Secondary objectives of these trials were to determine the
toxicities and pharmacokinetics of human leukocyte interferon. The
primary dose-limiting toxicity for intramuscular injection was
anorexia and weight loss. In the two trials involving 40 patients,
76% lost > 1 kg in weight (Table V). Fever which usually occurred in
only the first few days, was not dose-limiting. Dry mouth and
decreased secretions may have contributed to a possible interferon-
related death in a 64-year old woman with biopsy-proven pleural and
pulmonary tumor and interstitial fibrosis. When interferon was
started, she was hypoxic with a PO_2 of 68. Within the first three
weeks of interferon administration, she complained of dry eyes, dry
mouth and thick respiratory secretions; she required intubation and
was started on combination chemotherapy for her breast carcinoma.
She died of leukopenic sepsis 41 days after initiation of the
chemotherapy program. No such respiratory complication has been
reported in other patients receiving interferon for viral or
neoplastic disease.

One unexpected development was the appearance of clinical signs
and symptoms of herpes simplex virus infection in six of the patients
within a few days of initiation of interferon treatment. One patient
had an increase in herpes simplex virus complement fixation titer.

In these trials escalating doses from three million units to
nine million units did not result in significant increases in
systemic toxicities of buffy coat interferons. No further increase
in fever, weight loss or other parameters occurred. In terms of
labortory parameters, granulocytopenia (median white blood count
decrease from 5.9 x 10^9/liter to 3.1 x 10^9/liter) and mild SGOT
elevations (abnormal to start in 10% of patients, but abnormal in 50%
after treatment - a preinterferon range of 4 to 98 and

TABLE V

Phase II Evaluation of Human Leukocyte Interferon
in Metastatic Breast Carcinoma

	Patients with Toxicity (n = 40)					
	Abnormal Values[*] (%)		Range of Values[**]		Median[**]	
	pre IFN	post IFN	pre IFN	post IFN	pre IFN	post IFN
White blood count	8	68	1.9-19.2	1.9-10.8	5.9	3.1
Weight loss	-	76	-	-11.8-+1.5	-	-3.1
SGOT	10	50	4-98	13-242	21	39

[*]   wbc < 4 or > 12 x 10^9/1; weight loss > 1 kg; SGOT > 40
[**] wbc x 10^9/1; weight loss in kg; SGOT in international units

post-interferon range of 13 to 242) occurred (Table V). These
abnormalities were not more severe at the increased dose.

    Serum levels of interferons varied widely between patients. The
mean serum levels on day one at two, six and 24 hr following the
administration of three million units were 25, 50 and barely
measurable at 24 hr. However there was a wide range in terms of
individual values (peak titers at six hr varied from 0 to 208 units
after a dose of 3 x 10^6 units). With dose escalations from three to
nine million units, there was at least a three-fold escalation
achieved in terms of interferon titers.

    Secondary objectives also included correlation of disease
response with toxicities and with the immunological effects of
interferons. The data from the M.D. Anderson trial and the American
Cancer Society trial, when combined, suggested a correlation between
granulocyte nadir and disease response. Of those patients with a
granulocyte count of less than 1.5 x 10^9/liter, nine of 20 responded,
whereas of those patients with a granulocyte count that stayed above
1.5 x 10^9/liter, only three out of 23 responded (P = < 0.02). It is
interesting to note that four of six women who developed herpes
labialis responded, whereas only eight responded of the group of 34
who did not. This correlation with herpes labialis, while
significant, must be interpreted with caution because of the small
numbers in the response group. Age also correlated with response.
Both independently and when the results of the American Cancer
Society and M.D. Anderson trials were combined, older patients were

more likely to respond to interferon administration. Mean age of the
responding patients was 62, with a median of 64; the mean and median
for non-responders was 54 and 52 (< 0.01).

Spontaneous cell cytotoxicity (NK cell) and antibody-dependent
cell cytotoxicity (K cell) levels were determined in the nine
patients treated at the University of Wisconsin. Significant
increases in NK and K cell function occurred (Figure 1). Almost all
of the patients had augmented spontaneous cell-mediated cytotoxicity
and antibody-dependent cell-mediated cytotoxicity 48 hr after the
administration of the interferon. This enhancement gradually
declined, however, despite continued administration of interferon.
Off therapy, all patients returned to their baseline levels. Beta-2
microglobulin is a protein that is expressed by all cells and has
significant sequence homology with the constant portion of IgG.
Although its exact function is unknown, it is probably important in
HLA antigen expression on the surface of different types of cells.
In the University of Wisconsin patients, there was a very significant
elevation of beta-2 microglobulin following the initiation of
interferon treatment. At days 15 and 22, only one patient did not
have an increased level. To determine the specificity of this
effect, we evaluated a group of 16 women with metastatic breast
carcinoma who were getting cytotoxic chemotherapy. In these women no
elevation of beta-2 microglobulin occurred. Although the numbers of
patients were very small, these immunologic changes were not
correlated with disease response.

In summary, the clinical trials in breast carcinoma with buffy
coat interferon (alpha) produced in Helsinki, resulted in objective
partial regressions of established breast carcinoma (95% confidence
interval for true response frequency: 15 - 38%). Responses were
observed at four different institutions. Dose, route, schedule and
duration of administration, or interferon α subtype for optimal
effect were not defined. However, responses of longer duration
resulted from continued administration. The limiting toxicity of
daily intramuscular administration was anorexia and malaise. Neither
response nor toxicity was clearly dose-related over a three-fold
range. There was substantial individual variability of up to 100-
fold in serum interferon levels between patients. The mean peak
level was 60 units/dl. With the three-fold dose escalation, serum
levels increased proportionately and were more sustained. NK and K
cell levels increased initially and then declined, despite the
continued administration of interferon. Sustained increases in
beta-2 microglobulin also occurred.

Interferons are different antitumor compounds from those
currently in clinical use (Gresser, 1977; Vilcek et al., 1980; Borden
and Ball, 1981). However, clinical doses and schedules in breast
carcinoma have been largely to date empirically derived. Trials are
only now beginning to define a maximally tolerated dose of

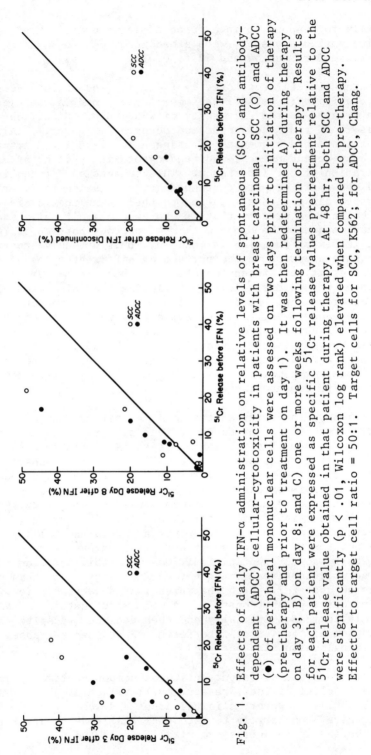

Fig. 1. Effects of daily IFN-α administration on relative levels of spontaneous (SCC) and antibody-dependent (ADCC) cellular-cytotoxicity in patients with breast carcinoma. SCC (○) and ADCC (●) of peripheral mononuclear cells were assessed on two days prior to initiation of therapy (pre-therapy and prior to treatment on day 1). It was then redetermined A) during therapy on day 3; B) on day 8; and C) one or more weeks following termination of therapy. Results for each patient were expressed as specific 51Cr release values pretreatment relative to the 51Cr release value obtained in that patient during therapy. At 48 hr, both SCC and ADCC were significantly (p < .01, Wilcoxon log rank) elevated when compared to pre-therapy. Effector to target cell ratio = 50:1. Target cells for SCC, K562; for ADCC, Chang.

recombinant and lymphoblastoid interferons. For rational design of continuing trials, biologically active doses in addition to clinically effective doses will need to be elucidated. The therapeutic activity of interferon α subtypes, which constitute the buffy coat interferon preparation, must be determined. Once optimal dose and schedule are determined, prospectively randomized trials will be required to define the therapeutic role of interferons. Such Phase III studies will compare effectiveness of interferons either alone or, as suggested by experimental studies, in combination with other modalities (Gresser et al., 1978; Chirigos and Pearson, 1973; Ortaldo and McCoy, 1980) for treatment of breast carcinoma.

REFERENCES

Balkwill, F., Watling, D., and Taylor-Papadimitriou, J. 1978, Inhibition by lymphoblastoid interferon of growth of cells derived from the human breast, Int. J. Cancer, 22:258.

Balkwill, F., Taylor-Papadimitriou, J., Fantes, K.H., and Sebesteny, A. 1980, Human lymphoblastoid interferon can inhibit the growth of human breast cancer xenografts in athymic (nude) mice. Eur. J. Cancer, 16:569.

Borden, E.C., and Ball, L.A. 1981, Interferons: biochemical, cell growth inhibitory, and immunological effects, Prog. Hematol., 12:299.

Borden, E.C., Gutterman, J.U., Holland, J.F., and Dao, T.L. 1981, Interferons in breast carcinoma: design and background leading to the American Cancer Society Program, in: "The Biology of the Interferon System", pp.391, E. DeMaeyer, G. Galasso, and H. Schellekens, eds., Elsevier/North Holland Biomedical Press, Amsterdam.

Borden, E.C., Holland, J.F., Dao, T.L., Gutterman, J.U., Wiener, L., Chang, Y-C., and Patel, J. 1982, Leukocyte-derived interferon (α) in human breast carcinoma, Ann. Int. Med., 97:1.

Came, P.E., and Moore, D.H. 1972, Effect of exogenous interferon treatment on mouse mammary tumors, J. Natl. Cancer Inst., 48:1151.

Cantell, K., Hirvonen, S., Morensen, K.E., and Phyälä, L. 1973, Human leukocyte interferon: production, purification, stability and animal experiments in the production and use of interferon for the treatment and prevention of human virus infection, in: "Proceedings of a Tissue Culture Association Workshop", C. Waymouth, ed., In vitro Monography, 3:35.

Chirigos, M.A., and Pearson, J.W. 1973, Cure of murine leukemia with drug and interferon treatment, J. Natl. Cancer Inst., 51:1367.

Gresser, I. 1977, On the varied biologic effect of interferon, Cellular Immunol., 34:406.

Gresser, I., Maury, C., and Tovey, M. 1978, Efficacy of combined interferon cyclophosphamide therapy after diagnosis of lymphoma in AKR mice, Eur. J. Cancer, 14:97.

Gutterman, J.U., Blumenschein, G.R., Alexanian, R., Yap, H-Y.,
    Buzdar, A.U., Cabanillas, F., Hortobagyi, G.N., Hersh, E.M.,
    Rasmussen, S.L., Harmon, M., Kramer, M., and Pestka, S. 1980,
    Leukocyte interferon-induced tumor regression in human
    metastatic breast cancer, multiple myeloma, and malignant
    lymphoma, Ann. Int. Med., 93:399.
Ortaldo, J.R., and McCoy, J.L. 1980, Protective effects of interferon
    in mice previously exposed to lethal irradiation, Rad. Res.,
    81:262.
Strander, H., Adamson, V., Aparisi, T., Broström, L.A., Cantell, K.,
    Einhorn, S., Hall, K., Ingimarsson, S., Nilsonne, U., and
    Söderberg, G. 1978, Adjuvant interferon treatment of
    osteosarcoma, Recent Results Cancer Res., 68:40.
Vilcek, J., Gresser, I., and Merigan, T. 1980, Regulatory functions
    of interferons, Annals NY Acad. Sci., 350:1.

LUNG CANCER

KARIN MATTSON AND LARS R. HOLSTI

Departments of Pulmonary Diseases and Radiotherapy and
Oncology, Helsinki University Central Hospital
Haartmaninkatu 4, 00290 Helsinki 29, Finland

Lung cancer is the leading cause of cancer death in men and in
some countries already the second leading cause of cancer death in
women. The incidence of the disease is still rapidly increasing in
women, while a levelling off may be taking place in men. The overall
five year survival has not improved significantly in the past 30
years and remains less than 10 per cent.

Ninety-five per cent of lung cancers are bronchogenic carcinomas
arising from the bronchial or bronchioloalveolar surface epithelium
or from bronchial mucous glands. The four major cell types are
epidermoid or squamous cell carcinoma (35-50 per cent), adenocarcinoma (20-40 per cent), large cell carcinoma (5 per cent) and
small cell carcinoma (20-25 per cent). These cell types differ with
respect to natural history and response to therapy. For this reason
lung cancer should be be referred to as one disease when therapeutic
aspects are discussed. For practical purposes of treatment,
bronchogenic carcinomas are divided into two main groups: non-small
cell (NSLC) and small cell (SCLC) carcinomas. At the time of
diagnosis, the disease has spread to regional nodes or distant sites
in 75 per cent of all patients and is therefore incurable by
traditional single local modality treatment. Even though a combined
treatment approach including some form of systemic therapy has been
introduced at most centers, systemic control is usually not achieved
regardless of possible local control. Therefore, there is a need to
identify new effective systemic agents. The biologic features of
SCLC make it more amenable to chemotherapy than NSCL (Hansen, 1982).
However, in spite of recent chemotherapeutic advances SCLC remains
one of the most aggressive and lethal tumors known. The median
survival of intensively treated patients is only 12 months and the
two-year survival 10-20 per cent. This is partly due to tumor

resistance to available drugs and/or radiation and partly to drug
toxicity.

EXPERIMENTAL BACKGROUND

Gresser's (1972, 1976) in vitro and in vivo studies indicated
that interferon (IFN) is not cytocidal but inhibits tumor cell multiplication and delays the rate of cell multiplication. SCLC cells
have short generation time and the marked cellular proliferation may
be accompanied by considerable cell loss. Any decrease or delay in
tumor cell proliferation and/or increase in tumor cell death may be
of therapeutic value. Schlag et al. (1982) showed that highly
purified fibroblast IFN did not significantly reduce colony forming
tumor growth of three human lung carcinomas. Studies with animal
models suggest that IFN doses higher than those given in current
clinical trials will be necessary to obtain a definitive beneficial
effect in man. IFN treatment in mice inoculated with Lewis lung
carcinoma resulted in a marked delay in the growth of the primary
tumor and in inhibition of the development of pulmonary metastases.
However, the dose required to obtain this effect was one-hundred to
one-thousand times larger than those which generally have been used
in trials in man (20 mu/kg/day) (Gresser and Bourali-Maury, 1972).
This might to some extent elucidate why only minor antitumor activity
was found in clinical trials where low-dose IFN was given for short
periods of time.

CLINICAL STUDIES

Non-small Cell Carcinoma of the Lung

Only one study has been reported. Fourteen previously treated
patients with measurable inoperable NSCLC were treated with low-dose
human leukocyte IFN (P-IF) 3×10^6 IU/day intramuscularly for 30 days
(Stoopler et al., 1980). No objective response was obtained. Out of
11 evaluable patients six showed progressive disease (PD) and five
stable disease (SD) at the end of the IFN treatment and for at least
30 days thereafter. Nine had adenocarcinoma and two epidermoid
carcinoma. The natural killer cell activity was significantly
increased in seven serially tested patients.

Small Cell Carcinoma of the Lung

Bleehen et al. (1982) studied the antitumor effect of single
agent high-dose human lymphoblastoid (HLBI) interferon (50 - 100 x
10^6 IU/m^2 daily) given as a continuous intravenous infusion for five
days followed by low-dose intramuscular maintenance therapy for three
weeks in previously untreated patients with SCLC. The patients were
subsequently submitted to conventional chemo-radiotherapy. Even

though the induction dose of HLBI in this study was fairly high, was
the total dose of IFN low and the total duration of IFN treatment
short. No tumor regression was observed during the treatment period
(8 SD; 2 PD) or one month after the completion of treatment (two SD;
six PD; two failed to complete treatment). The authors felt that IFN
as a single agent was unlikely to play a role in the treatment of
SCLC and that its toxicity was considerable. Toxicity included
fever, anorexia and weight loss, mild myelosuppression, severe
debility and in two patients the development of an inappropriate ADH
syndrome. However, in the final judgement of the value of IFN in
SCLC data on relapse pattern, outcome of other subsequent treatments
and survival should also be taken into consideration.

A similar study using high-dose human leukocyte interferon in
previously untreated patients with limited SCLC is currently carried
out by our group at the Helsinki University Central Hospital (Mattson
et al., 1982). Patient intake began in September 1981. Because in
some experimental tumor models, interferon inhibits the progression
of metastatic dissemination rather than eliminates the primary tumor
bulk (Gresser et al., 1976), we decided to test the efficacy of
prolonged low-dose maintenance treatment with IFN in combination with
radiotherapy in preventing subclinical systemic tumor growth in
addition to measuring the antitumor effect at the primary tumor site
of single high-dose intravenous IFN.

So far, six patients have received partially purified human
leukocyte IFN (P-IF B and A, specific activity 1-3 x 10^6 IU/mg
protein) and two have received highly purified IFN (NK2-IFN, specific
activity 1.2 x 10^8 IU/mg protein) obtained by passage through a
monoclonal antibody affinity chromatography column (NK2 Sepharose,
Celltech, England). The dose planned to be administered on days one
and two was 100 x 10^6 IU/24 hr, followed by 200 x 10^6 IU/24 hr on
days three - five, or a total of 800 x 10^6 IU/5 days as continuous
intravenous infusion. The intravenous treatment was followed by
low-dose maintenance treatment: 6 x 10^6 IU given intramuscularly
three times weekly, commencing on day eight. In case of locoregional
progression alone or isolated CNS relapse radiotherapy was given
while IFN treatment was continued until systemic non-CNS relapse,
when conventional combination chemotherapy was started. IFN is
unlikely to have an effect on CNS metastases because of the strong
blood-CNS barrier to IFN (Habif et al., 1975).

The mean duration of treatment with IFN alone was 18 weeks
(range 5-42), and with IFN plus concomitant radiotherapy 25+ weeks
(range 5-42+). Using the WHO criteria for evaluation of tumor
responses we found no objective response (Table I) but in three out
of eight patients tumor shrinkage was measured with a maximum area
reduction occuring at 16, 18 and 22 weeks of IFN single treatment.
The "response" lasted five, seven and 20 weeks calculated from the
day the maximum response had occurred. IFN thus seems to induce

TABLE I

Results of Treatment of SCLC with Human Leukocyte Interferon

Pat.	Total dose of IFN x 10^6 I.U.		Maximal response	Duration of response weeks	Site of progression
V.S.	878	P-IF	SD	5	Primary site
T.E.	1024	"	MR*	20	CNS
H.A.	1208	"	MR	25	-**
E.B.	1085	"	MR	42	Primary site
A.T.	650	"	SD	10	Primary site
A.W.	974	"	SD	10	Primary site
A.N.	902	NK2IFN	SD	7	Primary site
H.V.	938	"	SD	18	CNS

* 49% area reduction; ** IFN treatment stopped because of side effects;
SD stable disease; MR minimal response.

tumor shrinkage very gradually and very slowly. The greatest reduction in size (49 per cent area reduction) was measured from serial CT scans of a $T_2N_2M_0$ central tumor located in the left upper lobe bronchus. Five patients had SD for five - 18 weeks as calculated from the start of treatment. As the first site of disease relapse five patients showed locoregional progression alone after five - 42 weeks and two isolated CNS relapses after 18 and 20 weeks of single IFN. We feel that these promising results might be due to the differences in duration of treatment and/or in the interferon types used.

Split-course radiation therapy (30 Gy in 10 F - three weeks rest - 25 Gy in 10 F) to the primary tumor, the mediastinum and supra-clavicular nodes following and concomitant with IFN therapy induced exceptionally rapid tumor shrinkage in six out of seven patients. One patient (A.W.) died with disseminated disease and local relapse 20 weeks from the start of IFN treatment, or one month following radiotherapy to the primary site and to the brain. This patient refused any treatment during one month prior to death. Clinically severe radiation pneumonitis occured in four of six evaluable patients, two of whom (A.T., H.A.) died of acute hemoptysis ten and

25 weeks from the start of IFN therapy, or five and 50 days following radiotherapy. Autopsy revealed no macroscopic or microscopic tumor at any site but severe radiation pneumonitis.

Recently potentiation of radiation injury by IFN was shown in culture of Swiss 3T3 cells when mouse IFN was given two hours prior to irradiation (Dritschilo et al., 1982). This would be in accordance with our clinical findings in SCLC. On the other hand, it has also been demonstrated that a single intraperitoneal injection of 30,000 IU of mouse IFN administered one day following a LD_{100} dose irradiation significantly prolonged the mean survival time of mice, suggesting a radioprotective action of IFN (Ortaldo and McCoy, 1980). It seems important carefully to monitor dosage and timing of combinations of IFN and radiotherapy in order to avoid possibly excessive normal tissue damage and to optimize the therapeutic benefit of this combination.

Only two out of, at present, five potential patients have received chemotherapy subsequent to IFN-radiotherapy. One (V.S.) died 52 weeks after the start of IFN. Disseminated disease and local relapse were confirmed by autopsy. One (T.E.) is alive with disease at 40 weeks. The three remaining patients are alive at 37 weeks without disease (A.N.), and at 28 (H.V.) and 48 (E.B.) weeks with stable disease. Considering the very aggressive nature of SCLC with its tendency to rapid and early dissemination, our results are suggestive of a growth-delaying effect of IFN.

Fever with severe tremor during the peaks, malaise and muscle pain occurred in all patients throughout the five days of intravenous treatment. On the second day of the infusion a progressive mental and motor slowing set in. Great fatigue, somnolence, lack of initiative and loss of smell and taste were characteristic. Speech became unclear and inaccurate, and only slow answers could be obtained. Serial EEG recordings showed progressive general slowing of background activity from alpha to theta range with diffuse delta waves predominantly in the frontal lobe. Derangement of peripheral nervous function was revealed by slowing of motor and sensory conduction velocities on ENMG's.

Only with the high intravenous dose ($100-200 \times 10^6$ IU/24 hr) did CSF contain measurable amounts of IFN (35-110 IU/ml). Differential cell counts showed that an increase in the proportion of enlarged lymphocytes in CSF coincided with EEG abnormalities.

The neurophysiologic and clinical abnormalities gradually subsided within two - four weeks after the end of the high-dose phase while low-dose IFN treatment was continued. Side-effects with partially purified and with highly purified IFN were indistinguishable. Thus, the observed neurologic effects were probably caused by interferon and not by impurities in the IFN preparations. These observations suggest that adverse neurologic effects are a dose-limiting factor in high-dose IFN treatment.

Recently Started Clinical Trials

A randomized study for the evaluation of low-dose maintenance
interferon following chemo-radiotherapy induction in previously
untreated patients with SCLC is currently in progress at the Helsinki
University Central Hospital. A phase II investigation of low-dose
human leukocyte IFN in patients with SCLC who have relapsed after or
failed to respond to frontline therapy was initiated in 1982 at the
MD Anderson Hospital, Houston, Texas. At the same institution human
luekocyte IFN frontline therapy is under investigation since 1982 in
bronchoalveolar carcinoma, a subtype of adenocarcinoma. We are not
aware at present of any clinical studies under way with fibroblast
IFN or recombinant IFN in human lung cancer.

FINAL REMARKS

On the basis of the scanty information available today on IFN
treatment of lung cancer, it seems justifiable to put forward the
following tentative statements, which further studies may prove or
disprove. High doses of IFN and a small tumor burden may be factors
enhancing IFN efficacy, as suggested by the mouse experiments with
Lewis lung carcinoma and other transplantable tumors (Gresser, 1972;
Gresser et al., 1976). Long-term low-dose interferon may increase
the metastasis-free interval. Such an effect seems compatible with
our observations in SCLC patients and is suggested also by a
non-randomized study of IFN as adjuvant treatment in patients with
osteosarcoma (Strander, 1977). Potentiation of radiation injury by
IFN may occur and calls for careful patient monitoring as well as
timing of IFN and radiotherapy in order to avoid possible excessive
damage to normal tissue (Dritschilo et al., 1982) and to benefit from
possible synergism.

At present, the number of lung cancer patients treated with IFN
is too small to permit any conclusions as to whether IFN will be a
clinically useful drug against SCLC or NSCLC. More studies are
needed to evaluate the effects of different interferons, the dose and
route of administration and the treatment duration. It is
conceivable, however, that the immunomodulatory and antiproliferative
actions of interferons may offer possibilities for the future
development of combined schedules with IFN and conventional methods
reducing the tumor burden.

REFERENCES

Bleehen, N.M., Jones, D.H., and Slater, A.J. 1982, High dose human
    lymphoblastoid interferon in the treatment of small cell
    carcinoma of bronchus, in: "The III World Conference on Lung
    Cancer, Abstracts", May 17-20, 1982, p.161, Tokyo, Japan.

Dritschilo, A., Mossman, K., Gray, M., and Sreevalsan, T. 1982,
    Potentiation of radiation injury by interferon, Am. J. Clin.
    Oncol., 5:79.
Gresser, I. 1972, Anti-tumor effects of interferon, Advanc. Cancer
    Res., 16:97.
Gresser, I., and Bourali-Maury, C. 1972, Inhibition by interferon
    preparations of a solid tumor and pulmonary metastases in mice,
    Nature New Biol., 236:78.
Gresser, I., Maury, C., and Tovey, M. 1976, Interferon and murine
    leukemia. VII. Therapeutic effect of interferon preparations
    after diagnosis of lymphoma in AKR mice. Int. J. Cancer,
    17:647.
Habif, D.V., Lipton, R., and Cantell, K. 1975, Interferon crosses
    blood-cerebrospinal fluid barrier in monkeys, Proc. Soc. Exp.
    Biol. Med., 149:287.
Hansen, H.H. 1982, Management of small-cell anaplastic carcinoma,
    1980-1982, in: "Lung Cancer 1982", S. Ishikawa, Y. Hayata, and
    K. Suemasu, eds., Excerpta Medica, Amsterdam-Oxford-Princeton.
Mattson, K., Niiranen, A., Holsti, L.R., Iivanainen, M., Bergström,
    L., Standertskjöld-Nordenstam, C.G., Tarkkanen, J., Färkkilä,
    M., Anderson, L., Holsti, P., Kauppinen, H.-L., and Cantell, K.
    1982, High-dose human leukocyte interferon given as a five day
    continuous intravenous infusion followed by low-dose intra-
    muscular maintenance treatment in previously untreated patients
    with small cell carcinoma of the lung. Preliminary results,
    Eur. J. Resp. Dis. Suppl., 125:63:41.
Schlag, P., Schreml, W., and Herfarth, Ch. 1982, Effect of fibroblast
    interferon (IF-B) on colony forming tumor growth of
    miscellaneous carcinomas, in: "Proceedings of 13th International
    Cancer Congress", Sept. 8-15, 1982, p.243, Seattle, Washington.
Stoopler, M.B., Krown, S.E., Gralla, R.J., Cunningham-Rundles, S.,
    Stewart, W.E., and Oettgen, H.F. 1980, Phase II trial of human
    leukocyte interferon in non-small cell lung cancer, in: "II
    World Conference on Lung Cancer, Abstracts", June 9-13, 1980,
    p.221, Copenhagen.
Strander, H. 1977, Interferons: antineoplastic drugs? Blut, 35:277.

GASTROINTESTINAL CANCER

JOHN R. NEEFE

Divisions of Medical Oncology and Immunologic Oncology
Lombardi Cancer Research Center and Department of
Medicine, Georgetown University, Washington, D.C., U.S.A.

Gastrointestinal malignancy constitutes a major public health
problem with significant morbidity and mortality. The use of
interferon in this group of disorders is increasing, but for the most
part has been limited to colon cancer. Other gastrointestinal
malignancies are less common and generally involve disease which is
difficult to measure and, therefore, difficult to study.

Colorectal cancer is one of the leading causes of cancer
mortality. Over 100,000 new cases of colorectal cancer appeared in
the United States in 1981, and almost half of these individuals will
have died of this disease (American Cancer Society, 1981). Those
patients whose cancer has spread beyond the confines of the primary
tumor almost invariably die of the disease. No curative therapy is
available for the patient with metastatic disease; progress in the
therapy of colon cancer has come nearly to a halt with the
achievement of optimal surgical management of the early, resectable
case.

The primary therapeutic modality available for the patient with
advanced cancer of the colon consists of chemotherapy with 5-
fluorouracil. This drug has been widely used since its introduction
in 1957, and an immense experience has established that 20-25% of
patients will have tumor regression when treated with this agent.
Not only do the great majority of patients fail to respond to
5-fluorouracil, but for those who do respond, the response usually
lasts only a few months and may not translate either into improved
quality of life or into an increased duration of survival. No other
anti-cancer drug, nor any other modality of anti-cancer therapy, has
thus far proven superior to 5-fluorouracil in the palliation of
cancer of the colon, despite extensive investigations of numerous

approaches effective in other cancers.   Thus, the need for new
concepts and approaches to the management of disseminated cancer of
the colon is self-evident.

        In ideal circumstances, a trial of interferon as therapy in
patients with a particular malignancy would devolve from 1) an
understanding of the mechanism of anti-tumor activity of interferon,
2) evidence that this mechanism applies to the cancer at issue, and
3) evidence that this mechanism would be effective in confronting
tumors of an extent or stage likely to be encountered in the patient
trial.

        The mechanism of action of interferon as an antiviral and anti-
neoplastic agent has been the subject of numerous investigations for
some years now and this work has been reviewed extensively.
Currently, attention is focussed on 2,5A polymerase as a likely
pathway for explaining the antiviral activity of interferon,
particularly with regard to RNA viruses.   The polymerase is activated
by double stranded RNA unique to viral replication and, in turn, it
activates an endonuclease which cleaves the viral RNA (Baglioni,
1979; Farrell et al., 1978).   This mechanism is not easily extended
to colon cancer since evidence for a viral etiology is lacking.
There is some evidence that fibroblast interferon may kill a human
cell line HT-29 derived from an adenocarcinoma of the colon, although
the cell line was considered relatively resistant to this inhibition
(Ito and Buffet, 1981).

        It has been known for some time that interferon can influence
strongly the regulatory circuits in the immune system.   Immunological
forces are capable of discriminating foreign tissues including some
model tumors from normal tissues and they are capable of destroying
substantial concentrations of neoplastic tissue.   Attention has been
focussed on the various mediators of "natural resistance" including
natural killers, which destroy susceptible tumor targets bearing
certain widely represented antigenic specificities; K cells, which
destroy tumor targets coated by antibody; and monocytes/macrophages,
which inhibit the growth of susceptible tumors.   Interferon can
augment the activity of each of these modalities both _in vitro_ and _in
vivo_ (Herberman and Ortaldo, 1981).   There is substantial indirect
evidence which permits the inference that these activities could
mediate biologically significant tumor resistance in man, but there
is, as yet, no direct or conclusive proof of this proposition.
Certainly, there is no direct evidence that "natural resistance" or
interferon-augmented "natural resistance" inhibits colon cancer _in
vivo_.   It is of interest that tumor cell lines resistant to the anti-
proliferative effects of interferon in culture, may nevertheless be
susceptible to interferon-induced natural killing (Gresser and
Brouty-Boye, 1972; Chen et al., 1981).

        Tumor immunologists have demonstrated that immunological
mechanisms presently understood are effective against very early and

small tumors. There are very few examples in the literature of immunological control of model tumors proportionately as extensive as the tumors of the typical patient with advanced colon cancer. Obviously, cytotoxic chemotherapy is similarly more effective against small tumor burdens, and this realization has led to the combination of "debulking" procedures with chemotherapy of proven curative potential in such cancers as testicular, oat cell of the lung, and ovarian. Nevertheless, the complexity of immunoregulatory circuits and the possibilities of "down-regulation" or blockades by soluble antigen or antigen-antibody complexes and the possibility of suppression make the consideration of tumor bulk especially important in the administration of a potential immune modulator such as interferon to patients with advanced colon cancer.

Given these limits to the experimental basis for the use of interferon in advanced cancer, what rationale can be brought forward for clinical trials in our present state of knowledge? Firstly, there is the magnitude of the need. Colon cancer kills tens of thousands yearly and there is no truly effective therapy for the advanced case. Secondly, there is the consideration that half of colon cancer patients, those with limited disease amenable to surgery, are cured. However, many of those receiving surgery with curative potential subsequently relapse with incurable disease. The potential application of interferon in this "adjuvant" setting of the high-risk patient is extremely important. Traditionally, it has not been possible to mount adjuvant trials of new agents until substantial activity of the agent has been demonstrated in advanced disease. Since the ultimate role of interferon in colon cancer seems most likely to be as an adjuvant to surgical therapy of early disease, it is important to obtain any evidence of activity in advanced disease.

Most important as a basis for trial of interferon in advanced colon cancer, is the observation of response in chemotherapy-resistant colon cancer patients receiving interferon in phase I trials where a primary objective was the delineation of toxicity (Table I).

Hoffmann-La Roche sponsored extensive phase I trials of its clone A alpha interferon. One patient with colon cancer treated at the Frederick Cancer Research Center showed a transient minor response (Sherwin et al., 1982). At Baltimore Cancer Research Center, one patient with colon cancer also had a minor response in the form of decreased liver size and this response persisted for several months after discontinuation of interferon at eight weeks (Leavitt et al., 1982).

Schering Plough Research Division also sponsored phase I trials of its very similar cloned alpha-2 interferon. One patient received weekly interferon in an escalating fashion from 10^6 to 100×10^6

TABLE I

Responses to Interferon in Colon Cancer

Type of Interferon	Dose and Schedule	Responses
Clone A Alpha	50 mU/m^2 3x/wk	1 MR
Clone A Alpha	10 mU 2x/daily	1 MR
Cloned Alpha-2	1 to 100 mU/wk	1 PR
Clone A Alpha	50 mU/m^2 3x/wk	1 PR
Cantell-type Alpha	3 mU daily	none
Cloned Alpha-2	50 mU/m^2 5x/wk	In progress

MR = less than 50% decrease in measurable disease
PR = more than 50% decrease in measurable disease

units. This patient had received a debulking procedure prior to
interferon but had a normal physical examination and computed
tomography of the abdomen one year after interferon (Stefan
Madajewicz, personal communication). Several full-scale phase II
trials designed to demonstrate efficacy of interferon in advanced
colon cancer have been initiated.

At the Vincent T. Lombardi Cancer Center at Georgetown
University two trials are nearing completion. The first employs the
clone A alpha interferon being developed by Hoffmann-La Roche and the
second employs the cloned alpha-2 interferon manufactured by Schering
Plough.

Twenty-one patients have been entered into the first trial
(Neefe et al., submitted). All had histologically documented,
measurable adenocarcinoma of the colon or rectum and all advanced
disease. Informed consent was obtained. None had received prior
chemotherapy for advanced disease, although four had received
adjuvant radiotherapy or chemotherapy followed by a documented
disease-free interval. The average age was 60 and all patients were
minimally symptomatic and ambulatory with an average initial
performance of 85 on the Karnofsky scale. 18 had liver metastases.
Clone A alpha interferon (Hu rIFN αA, Hoffmann La-Roche) was
administered in a dose of 50 million units/m thrice weekly intramuscularly. No escalation of dose was permitted, but de-escalation
to 50% and then to 10% dose was permitted for grade III toxicity on
the WHO scale. Therapy was continued for three months or until
objective progression of disease.

18 patients were evaluable for response. One patient chose to discontinue therapy after five doses because of fatigue. Another developed intracranial metastases after four weeks, and therapy was discontinued at this time. In one, respiratory distress developed and therapy was discontinued. Of the remaining patients, all but one showed progressive disease in three months or less; one patient showed, at three months, complete disappearance of multiple pulmonary nodules on chest X-ray and less than 50% decrease in size of hepatic nodules on radioisotopic liver scan. The pulmonary nodules reappeared after the fourth month of therapy, and interferon was discontinued.

Clone A interferon in this schedule was well tolerated, but dose adjustment was required in 13 of 20 patients receiving therapy for more than two weeks. The toxicities encountered were similar to those reported previously with clone A interferon (Gutterman et al., 1982). The most frequent causes for reduced doses of interferon included elevated hepatic enzymes, of which lactic dehydrogenase and the transaminases were representative, and fatigue.

Peak circulating levels of interferon of 996 to 5836 units/ml were detected usually at two - eight hours following intramuscular administration. Immunological monitoring was performed, and only preliminary data are available. These suggest that augmentation of natural killer activity and/or K cell activity occurred in most patients during the first three weeks. The effect was not persistent in those patients measured serially for thee months.

Another trial at the Vincent T. Lombardi Cancer Research Center at Georgetown University employs genetically engineered alpha-2 interferon (Schering Plough Research Division). This interferon, whose amino acid sequence is nearly identical to that of clone A interferon, is being administered in a dose of 50 million units/m^2 intravenously daily for five days. Each cycle is followed by a variable rest period of at least one week until full recovery from side effects. This schedule had been associated with responses in colon cancer patients in the phase I trial of alpha-2 interferon. Although the interferon is similar to that employed in the first trial described, the intermittent administration of a loading course represents a very significant distinction from the first trial in view of the possibility that the efficacy of interferon is highly dependent on schedule.

A third trial has been conducted and completed at UCLA. 18 evaluable patients, most heavily pretreated, received human leukocyte interferon at three million units per day, five days per week. The interferon was prepared by the New York Blood Bank from human buffy coat by the Cantell method. All patients progressed on therapy in a median time of five weeks (Figlin, in press).

Colon cancer is highly resistant to all forms of therapy, as has been demonstrated in literally hundreds of trials of many different agents over the past several decades. Taken in this context, the several responses to interferon reported thus far may be considered significant. On the other hand, it is clear that the particular interferons tested, when used at the doses and schedules employed, are not going to have dramatic impact upon the management of colon cancer. It is important to consider what generalizations can be made at present concerning the use of interferon in colon cancer.

Interferon is a complex material with more than a dozen native sequences known, and some of these sequences have only limited homology one to another. An additional structural complication is the unknown importance of glycosylation in the function of interferon.

Although the clone A interferon and alpha-2 interferon are known to have high levels of antiviral activity in human test systems and also have demonstrated at least some antitumor activity in human patients, the relative effectiveness of the various interferon sequences is very poorly understood at present. Secondly, it is only an assumption drawn from the usual experience with cytotoxic chemotherapy that high doses of interferon are desirable in treating cancer patients. The possibility that lower doses may be more "physiologic" must be considered. There is some evidence that less than maximal doses of some interferons may be more effective in augmenting in vivo immune responses. We (Bash et al., submitted) and others (Kariniemi et al., 1980) have observed a biphasic response of natural cytotoxicity against tumor targets, in which an early fall in activity is followed by a later rise. It must be considered possible that a schedule of daily or every other day administration may tend to abort the delayed rise. These considerations would raise the possibility that other doses and schedules of administration would result in much more effective immune modulation and much greater antitumor activity.

Finally, it should be understood that the true role of interferon may likely be in the adjuvant therapy of cancer. While experience tells us that effective adjuvants show substantial activity against advanced disease, there is no a priori logic for thinking this to be true of all agents or classes of agents. A problem with the adjuvant trial of interferon is the ethical difficulty in offering an experimental drug to a population of patients, some of whom will not recur even without therapy. In the case of interferon with colon cancer, a conservative resolution of the problems would dictate that adjuvant trials be reserved until a stronger basis for choosing the particular interferon and for choosing the dose and schedule may be developed. Nevertheless, there is sufficient evidence of activity of interferon in advanced colon cancer at the present time to encourage strong efforts to obtain this information which would allow an adjuvant trial to proceed.

REFERENCES

American Cancer Society 1981, Cancer Statistics, Cancer, J. Clin.,
    31:13.
Baglioni, C. 1979, Interferon-induced enzymatic activities and their
    role in the antiviral state, Cell, 17:255.
Bash, J.A., Teitelbaum, D., and Neefe, J.R. Immunomodulating
    activities of human leukocyte interferon in advanced cancer
    patients. Submitted.
Chen, H-Y, Sato, T., Fuse, A., Kuwata, T., and Content, J. 1981,
    Resistance to interferon of a human adenocarcinoma cell line
    HEC-1, and its sensitivity to natural killer cell action, J.
    Gen. Virol., 52:177.
Farrell, P.J., Sen, G.C., Dubois, M.F., et al. 1978, Interferon
    action: two distinct pathways for inhibition of protein
    synthesis by double-stranded RNA, Proc. Natl. Acad. Sci. USA,
    75:5893.
Figlin, R.A., Callaghan, M., and Sarna, G. Phase II trial of alpha
    (human leukocyte) interferon administered daily in
    adenocarcinoma of the colon/rectum. In press.
Gresser, I., and Brouty-Boye, D. 1972, On the mechanism of the
    antitumor effect of interferon in mice, Nature, 239:167.
Gutterman, J.U., Fein, S., and Quesada, J. 1982, Recombinant
    leukocyte A interferon: pharmokinetics, single dose tolerance,
    and biologic effects in cancer patients, Ann. Int. Med., 96:549.
Herberman, R.H., and Ortaldo, J.R., 1981, Natural killer cells: their
    role in defenses against disease, Science, 214:24.
Ito, M., Buffet, R.F. 1981, Cytocidal effect of purified fibroblast
    interferon on tumor cells in vitro, J. Natl. Cancer Inst.,
    66:819.
Kariniemi, A.L., Timonen, T., and Kousa, M. 1980, Effect of leukocyte
    interferon on natural killer cells in healthy volunteers.
    Scand. J. Immunol., 12:371.
Leavitt, R.D., Duffey, P.L., Wiernik, P.H., et al. 1982, Human
    leukocyte A interferon (IFL-rA) in: Proc. ASCO, 1:41.
Neefe, J.R., Fein, S., Smith, F.P., Harris, M., Silgals, R., Ayoob,
    M., and Schein, P.S. A phase II trial of recombinant human
    leukocyte A interferon (IFL-ra) colon cancer. Submitted.
Sherwin, S., Knost, J., Fein, S., et al. A multiple dose phase I
    trial of recombinant leukocyte A interferon in cancer patients,
    J. Amer. Med. Assoc. In press.

BRAIN TUMORS

SATOSHI UEDA, KIMIYOSHI HIRAKAWA, YOSHIO NAKAGAWA
KENZO SUZUKI AND TSUNATARO KISHIDA

Department of Neurosurgery and Microbiology
Kyoto Prefectural University of Medicine
Kyoto 602, Japan

INTRODUCTION

Interferon (IFN) is a humoral factor derived from cells after viral infection. It is known to be a protein which exerts non-specific antiviral activity in homologous cells through cellular metabolic processes involving synthesis of both RNA and protein. Recent extensive studies on IFN have revealed that it has other biological activities, including an antitumor effect. Since Gresser's (1970) study of IFN on experimental tumors and Strander's (1973, 1974) clinical trial on osteosarcoma patients have been reported, great expectation has been placed on IFN as an antitumor drug. However, because of difficulties in producing a sufficient amount of human IFN, the number of clinical studies has not been adequate to evaluate its effect against malignant brain tumors.

We administered IFN to patients with malignant brain tumors who had been taken off their usual treatment and investigated the effects of IFN on these tumors (Nakagawa, 1980; Ueda, 1982; Sawada, 1982; Hirakawa, 1982).

MATERIALS AND METHODS

Interferon

Human leukocyte interferon (Hu IFN-α) used in this study was obtained from the Green Cross Corporation and Kyoto Red Cross Blood Center in Japan. Its specific activity was over 10^6 IU/mg protein. It was kept frozen and dissolved by saline before clinical use.

Patients

Out of a total of 22 patients with primary or metastatic brain
tumor treated with IFN, 13 patients were selected to evaluate the
strict clinical potency of IFN; these patients did not receive
combination therpy with other anticancer drugs. The histological
classification of the surgical specimens were seven glioblastomas,
two medulloblastomas, one astrocytoma, one ependymoma and two
metastasis. The female to male ratio was seven:six; their ages
ranged from five to 66 years.

All patients underwent surgical removal of the tumors, followed
by ^{60}Co irradiation (5000 - 5500 rad). Some of them were given
additional chemotherapy with ACNU, procarbazine and vincristine after
irradiation. To exclude any effects of the previous treatment on the
tumors, IFN administration was started at least six months after
terminating the usual treatment; tumor recurrence was demonstrated
from signs and/or CT scan. IFN was given without other combination
therapy.

Interferon Administration

Two series of clinical studies of IFN were carried out: systemic
administration and local administration.

(a) Systemic administration. This group consisted of ten
patients. IFN was given by intramuscular injection into the gluteal
muscles for four to ten months. According to the dosage of IFN, they
were randomly divided into two subgroups, a low dosage group of six
cases and a high dosage group of four cases. The low dosage group
received 5×10^4 IU once a week and up to 3.4×10^6 IU totally. The
high dosage group received 3×10^6 IU every other day, up to 1.9×10^8
IU totally.

(b) Local administration. In four patients, IFN was given
locally through an Omaya reservoir which was placed on the bone flap;
the distal end of the tube was inserted into the dead space after the
brain tumors were removed. By percutaneous injection into this
device, IFN could be given directly into the tumor bed and the cyst
fluid or debris could be aspirated. These patients received 5 or 10
$\times 10^5$ IU daily or weekly up to 2.8×10^7 IU totally for one to six
months. Case four received the local treatment after he had failed
to respond to the general administration.

Evaluation of the Effects

General conditions, neurological signs and blood analysis were
monitored carefully. The immunological parameters such as photo-
hemaggulutinin (PHA) and purified protein derivatives of tuberculin
(PPD) skin test, pheripheral lymphocyte counts, Natural killer cell

TABLE I

Criteria for Estimating Responses

Response	Criteria
Complete Remission (CR)	Clinical and radiological improvement
Partial Remission (PR)	Clinical or radiological improvement
Unchanged (U)	No clinical and/or radiological changes
Worsened (W)	Clinical and/or radiological deterioration of the disease

(NK) activity (Herberman, 1979) using Hela cells as the target, and immunoglobulin of the patients were examined repeatedly before and after the treatment. The effects of IFN therapy on the brain tumor were evaluted by the changes of tumor volumes which were estimated by tracing the enhanced lesion on each slice of serial CT scans before and after the treatment, and converting these measurement to percentages which indicate the tumor volume as 100% just before the IFN treatment.

Analysis of cell kinetics using DNA cytofluorometry (Takamatsu, 1980; Suzuki, 1981) was also performed on the specimens taken during reoperations or autopsies to detect possible changes after IFN therapy.

The final evaluation of the clinical effects of IFN on the brain tumor patients was determined using the criteria which divided the results into four groups after the treatment (Table I).

RESULTS

General Condition of the Patients

Though some improvement in the patients general condition, after IFN treatment, such as good appetite, slight recovery of consciousness or increased daily activities was observed, it did not warrant a re-evaluation of one grade of the Karnofsky's performance scale. Thus these minimum effects could not be included into the final evaluation of the patients.

Side Effects

In four of the thirteen cases, transient fever (38-39°C) was
seen after IFN injection, but it was easily controlled with an
antipyretic. This transient attack of fever appeared to be the only
side effect caused by IFN. There were no remarkable changes in liver
or renal function; urinalysis and blood analysis were also normal.
In the local administration group, there were two cases of meningitis
which appeared to be caused by contamination during serial
injections; they recovered by the general and local administration of
antibiotics.

Immunological Parameters

No change in immunoglobulin level in serum was noted, but PHA
and PPD skin tests and peripheral lymphocyte counts showed some
transient improvement after IFN injection (Figures 1 and 2). The
changes seen were greater with systemic administration. NK cell
activity was also augmented as shown in Figure 3 by both systemic and
local administration.

Tumor Growth Curves

Figure 4 shows the tumor growth curves of cases one to five in
which IFN was administered systemically by intramuscular injection.
In cases one and two, a 50% decrease in tumor volume could be seen
after IFN treatment; before treatment, both cases had gradual curve

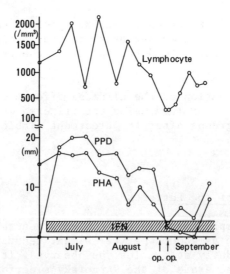

Fig. 1.   Changes of lymphocyte count in peripheral blood and PPD and
          PHA skin test of patient 4.

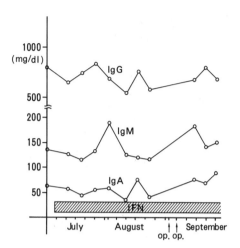

Fig. 2.   Changes of immunoglobulin level in serum of patient 4.

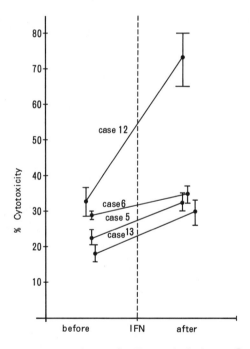

Fig. 3.   Showing augmentation of NK activities of patients 5 and 6
          (systemic administration) and patients 12 and 13 (local
          administration).

TABLE II

Systemic Administration of IFN

Case	Age	Sex	Tumor	Single Dose(IU)	Total Dose(IU)	Duration (M)	Side Effect	Response	Outcome
1	42	F	Glioblastoma	5×10^4 weekly	2.4×10^6	12	none	PR	alive 81M*
2	11	F	Medulloblast	5×10^4 weekly	3.4×10^6	17	none	PR	dead 54M
3	55	F	Glioblastoma	5×10^4 weekly	3.4×10^6	17	none	W	dead 28M
4	51	M	Glioblastoma	3×10^6 alt day	129×10^6	4	fever	W	dead 13M
5	17	F	Astrocytoma	3×10^6 alt day	191×10^6	17	fever	U	alive 42M
6	9	M	Mudulloblast	3×10^6 alt day	124.10^6	11	none	U	dead 40M
7	33	F	Glioblastoma	3×10^6 alt day	40×10^6	5	none	W	dead 34M
8	56	M	Glioblastoma	5×10^4 weekly	1.2×10^6	6	none	W	dead 16M
9	66	M	Metastasis	5×10^4 weekly	3.35×10^6	6	none	W	dead 12M
10	63	M	Metastasis	5×10^4 weekly	3.4×10^6	17	none	U	alive 32M

* M: Month

slopes. No effect on tumor growth could be seen in cases three, four
and five of which brain tumors had already shown rapid growth at the
time IFN administration was started.

Figure 5 shows the three cases in which IFN was given directly
into the tumor bed through the Omaya reservoir; one of the three
showed some decrease in tumor size after treatment but eventually
died.

Histological examination of the surgical or autopsy specimens
revealed no substantial difference before and after treatment.
Analysis of DNA content by cytofluorometry showed an increased ratio
of polyploid cells after IFN treatment. This might be related to the
growth inhibition seen on CT scans of the cases. The results are
tabulated in Table II (systemic administration) and Table III (local
administration).

DISCUSSION

The mechanism of the antitumor effect of IFN has been known with
regard to both the direct and indirect cytotoxicity. In order to
determine its clinical potency as an antitumor agent against brain
tumors, we administered IFN alone to primary and metastatic brain
tumor patients carefully evaluating their general and neurological
conditions, immunological parameters and tumor mass on CT scans, with
various dosages and routes. No other combination therapy was givn
during this period.

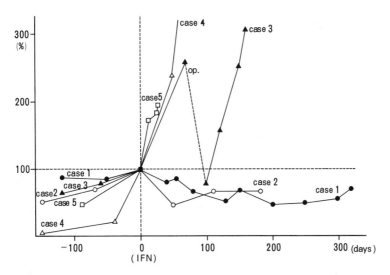

Fig. 4.   Tumor growth curves of patients 1 to 5 (systemic
          administration).

TABLE III

Local Administration

Case	Age	Sex	Tumor	Single Dose(IU)	Total Dose(IU)	Duration (M)	Side Effect	Response	Outcome
11	5	F	Ependymoma	1×10^6 weekly	8×10^6	2	fever	W	dead 41M
12	57	M	Glioblastoma	1×10^6 daily	25×10^6	1	fever	PR	dead 18M
13	41	F	Glioblastoma	1×10^6 daily	28×10^6	1	none	PR	alive 55M
14*	56	M	Glioblastoma	5×10^6 twice a week	4.5×10^6	1	none	W	dead 16M

* Was given local administration after failing to respond to general administration.
  (Case 8 in Table II)
  Cases 11 and 14 had meningitis during serial local injections.

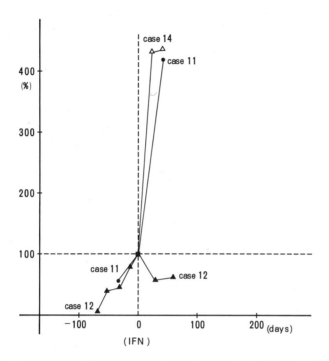

Fig. 5.   Tumor growth curves of patients 11, 12 and 14 (local
          administration).

Tumor mass can be easily measured by tracing the enhanced lesion
of each slice of serial CT before and after the treatment.   At
present, this appears to be the best method for accurately
determining the antitumor effect.

Upon systemic administration, two cases out of ten showed, 50%
decrease in tumor volume after IFN treatment, and these cases were
evaluated as partial remission according to our criteria.   However it
should be noted that both cases showed gradual growth curve slopes
before the treatment.   We could not see such a decrease when IFN was
started against the rapidly growing tumors as seen in cases three,
four and five.   These results appeared to be similar to those of
Merigan (1978) who reported that IFN was effective in inactive cases
but not in advancing cases of non-Hodgkin's lymphoma.

Upon local administration, two out of four cases showed partial
decrease in tumor volume, though one eventually died from tumor
regrowth.   Local administration can maintain a much higher concentration for a longer time than general administration.   From our
study, it could not be concluded whether local administration had a
superior antitumor effect than systemic administration.   Although

there are some reports of good results obtained by the intratumoral injection of IFN in patient with subcutaneous metastasis of neuro-blastoma (Sawada, 1979) and melanoma (Ishihara, 1982), there might have been other unknown factors besides the pharmacologic effect of IFN to account for those results.

Concerning the type of IFN and its antitumor effects, a recent study (Imanishi, 1981) has shown that there were no substantial differences in the magnitude of growth inhibition between human leucocyte, fibroblast and lymphoblastoid IFNs, though these findings are controversial. Nagai et al. (1982) reported good responses in treating brain tumors using HuIFN-β combined with radiochemotherapy, though they could not attribute the results to the effect of IFN alone. None of our thirteen cases treated with IFN alone achieved complete remission.

The host's cellular immune responses were augmented by IFN treatment. NK cells were also activated by the intracranial administration of IFN. NK activities showed interesting fluctuations during IFN treatment which will be reported later in detail.

From these clinical results, we conclude that IFN augmented the host's cellular immune reaction, and inhibited the growth of the slowly growing brain tumors, but it did not produce marked effect against rapidly growing tumors when administered systemically or locally.

However, there are still many problems to be studied. Dosage, route, interval and combination with other drugs need to be optimised. Further investigation is in progress from the both clinical and experimental aspects for IFN therapy of malignant brain tumors in our institute.

ACKNOWLEDGEMENTS

This research was supported in part by the research project grant-in-aid for scientific research 1981, No. 56470490, and by the grant-in-aid for cancer research 1981, No. 56010064, from the Ministry of Education of Japan.

REFERENCES

Gresser, I. and Bourali, C. 1970, Antitumor effect of interferon preparations in mice, J. Natl. Cancer Inst., 45:365.
Herberman, R.B., Ortaldo, J.R. and Bonnard, G.D. 1979, Augmentation by interferon of human natural and antibody dependent cellmediated cytotoxicity, Nature, 277:221.
Hirakawa, K., Ueda, S., Nakagawa, Y., Suzuki, K., Fukuma, S., Kita,

M., Imanishi, J. and Kishida, T. 1982, Effect of human leucocyte
interferon on malignant brain tumors, Cancer (in press).

Imanishi, J., Amagai, T., Pak, C.B., Oishi, K., Kawamura, H.,
Matsubara, M., Kita, M., Tanimoto, T. and Kishida, T. 1981,
Comparative studies on the inhibitory effect of human
interferons on the growth of tumor cells, J. Kyoto Pref. Univ.
Med., 90:409 (English Abstract).

Ishihara, K., Hayasaka, K. and Hasegawa, F. 1982, Treatment of
malignant melanoma by intratumoral administration of human
fibroblast interferon in: "The Clinical Potential of
Interferons", R. Kono and J. Vilcek, eds., University of Tokyo
Press, Tokyo.

Merigan, T.C., Sikora, K., Breeden, H., Levy, R. and Rosenberg, S.A.
1978, Preliminary observations on the effect of human leukocyte
interferon in non-Hodgkin's lymphoma, N. Engl. J. Med.,
299:1449.

Nagai, M., Arai, T., Kohno, S. and Kohase, M. 1982, Interferon
therapy for malignant brain tumors in: "The Clinical Potential
of interferons", R. Kono and J. Vilcek, eds., University of
Tokyo Press, Tokyo.

Nakagawa, Y., Kirakawa, K., Ueda, S., Suzuki, K., Kishida, T. and
Imanishi, J. 1980, Clinical trial of interferon for malignant
brain tumor, J. Kyoto Pref. Med., 118:749 (English Abstract).

Sawada, T., Toshihisa, F., Kusunoki, T., Imanishi, J. and Kishida, T.
1979, Preliminary report on the clinical use of human leucocyte
interferon in neuroblastoma. Cancer Treat. Rep., 63:2111.

Sawada, T., Tozawa, M., Kidowaki, T., Tanaka, T., Kusunoki, T.,
Nakagawa, Y., Suzuki, K., Ueda, S., Hirakawa, K., Oku, T., Kita,
M. and Kishida, T. 1982, Clinical use of human leucocyte
interferon in neurogenic tumors and other childhood tumors in:
"The Clinical Potential of Interferons", R. Kono and J. Vilcek,
eds., University of Tokyo Press, Tokyo.

Strander, H., Cantell, K., Carlstrom, G. and Jakobson, P. 1973,
Clinical and laboratory investigations on man: systemic
administration of potent interferon to man. J. Natl. Cancer
Inst., 51:733.

Strander, H., Cantell, K., Jakobsson, P.A., Nilsonne, U. and
Söderberg, G. 1974, Exogenous interferon therapy of osteogenic
sarcoma, Acta. Orthop. Scan., 45:958.

Suzuki, K., Yoshino, E., Ueda, S., Nakanishi, K., Nojou, Y., Fukuda,
M. and Hirakawa, K. 1981, Estimation of the prognosis of
malignant brain tumors - Volumetry by means of CT scanning and
DNA histogram. CT Research, 3:687 (English Abstract).

Takamatsu, T., Nakanishi, K., Onouchi, Z., Fukuda, M. and Fujita, S.
1980, Nonspecific ("Pseudoplasmal") dye binding in Feulgen
neclear staining and its blocking by azocarmin G.
Histochemistry, 66:169.

Ueda, S., Hirakawa, K., Suzuki, K., Nakagawa, Y., Ibayashi, N. and
Kishida, T. 1982, Interferon therapy for brain tumor patients.
Neurological Surgery (Tokyo), 10:49 (English Abstract).

BONE TUMORS

LARS-ÅKE BROSTRÖM AND ULF NILSONNE

Department of Orthopaedic Surgery, Karolinska Hospital
Stockholm, Sweden

INTRODUCTION

Primary bone tumors are uncommon lesions and it would seem that
interferon (IFN) therapy so far has been tried only in osteosarcoma.
Osteosarcoma is a malignant disease of bone mainly afflicting young
individuals with a predilection for the age group between 15 and 25
years. Its most common localization is the metaphyseal area of a
long bone. In about 70% of all cases osteosarcoma is situated near
the knee joint, i.e. in the distal femoral metaphysis, the proximal
tibia, or the fibular metaphysis. The incidence of the disease may
be estimated at approximately two cases per million inhabitants
annually (Broström, 1979; Cancer Treatment Reports, 1978; Dahlin and
Coventry, 1967). Like other primary malignant tumors of bone,
osteosarcoma is therefore a rare type of tumor. Centralized
management is consequently a prerequisite if a maximum of experience
is to be gained in the diagnosis and treatment of these patients, and
the Department of Orthopaedic Surgery at the Karolinska Hospital in
Stockholm serves as a referral center for more than half of all bone
tumor cases in Sweden.

Osteosarcoma is a highly malignant disease. Prior to 1970
overall survival was 10-20% (Cancer Treatment Reports, 1978; Dahlin
and Coventry, 1967). In 80% of cases pulmonary metastases developed
within one year. Treatment was a rule confined to irradiation and
radical surgery, often consisting in severely mutilating amputations,
which caused osteosarcoma patients to be labelled as hopeless and
tragic cases.

Such was the situation until the early 1970's, when the
possibility of a new approach was suggested by the experimental

141

studies on IFN pursued during the preceding decade. The antiviral
effect of IFN had become well-known, and there were some indications
to suggest that, in animals at least, osteosarcoma might be
virus-induced. Evidence had been brought forward that IFN had an
inhibitory effect on cell growth (Gresser, 1977; Paucker et al.,
1962), and subsequent studies had also demonstrated a marked
inhibitory effect on osteosarcoma cells in vitro (Strander and
Einhorn, 1977).

EXPERIMENTAL STUDIES

Several reports have shown that IFN's exert certain effects on
cell growth. Inhibitory effects on cell multiplication have been
demonstrated in both normal and tumor cells. Some cells are highly
sensitive, whereas others are more or less resistant (Gresser, 1977).
The mechanisms underlying growth inhibitory effects have been the
subject of intensive research disclosing that such effects on the
cells may be direct as well as indirect. IFN's have been described
in terms like "cell regulatory molecules" (Balkwill, 1979), and as
such their properties have been turned to account in the treatment of
malignant tumors in man.

Most of our knowledge of the antitumor effects of IFN's is
derived from studies on tissue culture systems and experimental
systems in animals with oncogenic viruses. Such studies have mainly
been based on the use of IFN-α and where bone tumors are concerned
they have been concentrated on osteosarcoma.

Osteosarcoma Cell Lines

Cell lines have been cultivated from different human
osteosarcomas and their sensitivity to HuIFN-α has been tested
(Chirigos and Pearson, 1973). Although some variations in
sensitivity have been found, clear dose-dependent growth inhibitory
effects of IFN could be demonstrated (Fig. 1). IFN in doses of
10-100 units per ml, which is equivalent to the serum levels found in
man after administration of 3×10^6 units, has been found to produce
a fairly strong inhibition of tumor cell growth. All osteosarcoma
cell lines tested retain their sensitivity to IFN and so far no
selection of IFN-resistant cells has been demonstrated (Strander and
Einhorn, 1977).

Studies on osteosarcoma cell lines have also provided
indications of tissue specificity. IFN-β has been demonstrated to
have a more pronounced growth inhibitory effect than IFN-α on
osteosarcoma cell lines, whereas the situation was reversed for
Burkitt lymphoma cell lines (Einhorn and Strander, 1977).

The combined effect of IFN and methotrexate on human
osteosarcoma cell lines has also been analyzed, but no synergistic,

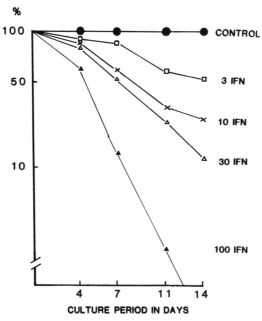

Fig. 1.   The inhibitory effect of Hu IFN-α on the osteosarcoma cell
line T$_2$56 grown as a monolayer culture in Eagles minimal
essential medium. Cell viability was determined by trypan
blue exclusion. The effect is expressed as the percentage
ratio of the number of living cells in the cultures containing IFN to the number of living cells found in simultaneously grown control cultures.

●———●	control	(medium only)
□———□	IFN 3	units/ml
×———×	IFN 10	units/ml
△———△	IFN 30	units/ml
▲———▲	IFN 100	units/ml

inhibitory or blocking effects on tumor cell growth could be detected
(Broström, 1980) (Fig. 2).

Transplantable Tumors

Reports on the antitumor effects of IFN on transplanted solid
human tumors in animals are sparse. In nude mice the IFN inducer
poly (I)-poly (C) has been reported to have an inhibitory effect on
fibrosarcoma (De Clercq et al., 1978) and IFN itself to inhibit the
growth of human breast cancer xenografts (Balkwill et al., 1980).
These experiments were performed with IFN-α and IFN-β.

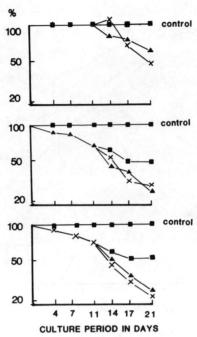

Fig. 2.   The effects of pretreatment with either Hu IFN-α or metho-
          trexate on the osteosarcoma cell line 393T.

          ■——■   control (medium only)
          x——x   IFN 10 units/ml
          ▲——▲   methotrexate 10 nM

        Experiments with murine osteosarcomas have shown that IFN
inhibits tumor growth and IFN-inducers such as Bru-Pel can enhance
host resistance to tumor growth (Glasgow et al., 1978; Glasgow et
al., 1979). One study reports IFN-γ to be a hundred-fold more
effective than IFN-α and active in very small doses in osteosarcoma
(Crane et al., 1978). From other experimental systems with murine
tumors it is evident that IFNs are most effective if the tumor load
is small, while additive effects have been reported with drugs such
as BCNU and cyclophosphamide (Chirigos and Pearson, 1973; Glasgow and
Kern, 1981; Gresser et al., 1978).

        Further experiments are required, however, to analyze the anti-
tumor effects on transplanted tumors of HuIFN of different kinds and
in various combinations, and perhaps in combination with other antitumor therapy.

CLINICAL INTERFERON TRIAL ON OSTEOSARCOMA PATIENTS
        Spurred by the results of the experimental studies Ulf Nilsonne
and Hans Strander at the Karolinska Hospital decided to test the

effect of IFN on osteosarcoma at the clinical level.   The conditions
for such a clinical trial were felt to be highly favorable,
particularly with respect to osteosarcoma, since the rapid progress
of this highly malignant disease would allow any response to
treatment to be registered rapidly.

The first patient was a young woman with an osteosarcoma
localized to the pelvis, a site which experience had shown to be
associated with an even poorer prognosis than for osteosarcoma in the
extremities (Dahlin and Coventry, 1967).   The tumor was removed by
local resection and IFN therapy initiated simultaneously.   One year
later the patient had no metastases or recurrence, thereby showing a
wholly different course of the disease than normally observed.   This
clearly warranted further testing of IFN therapy in cases of
osteosarcoma and initiated its first clinical trial in the treatment
of malignant disease (Strander et al., 1982).   The experience yielded
by this clinical trial furthermore triggered a rapidly growing
interest in IFN treatment for several other malignant conditions.

Starting in 1972, 51 patients with osteosarcoma have been
treated at the Section of Orthopedic Oncology at the Karolinska
Hospital.   The IFN group was made up of a consecutive series
consisting exclusively of patients with so-called primary classical
osteosarcoma, and consequently excluding periosteal, paraosteal or
irradiation-induced osteosarcomas.   Moreover, all patients with
demonstrable metastases at the time of diagnosis were excluded from
the series.   HuIFN-α produced by Cantell was used in a dose of three
million units injected intramuscularly, administered daily for one
month from the time of diagnosis, and thereafter three times weekly
for a total period of 1.5 years.   Only minor side effects were noted
and in no case IFN treatment had to be discontinued because of
adverse reactions (Ingimarsson et al., 1979).   Interferon was the
only adjuvant treatment in this patient series, and no chemotherapy
was given.

The patients in the IFN series not only received a new form of
adjuvant therapy, but surgical treatment too was considerably
modified in comparison with conventional earlier treatment.   In 17 of
the 51 cases, consequently, amputation could be avoided and was
replaced by radical local tumor resection (Nilsonne and Strander,
1981).   Reconstruction of the bone defects left by total or partial
joint resection was achieved by endoprosthetic replacement or massive
boen grafting (Fig. 3).

The results of this treatment were evaluated with the aid of two
control groups.   One group of a series of 35 so-called historical
controls, comprizing all osteosarcoma patients treated at the
Karolinska Hospital during the period 1952-1972 by the conventional
methods prevailing at that time, i.e. irradiation and ablative
surgery.   An additional control group was made up of "concurrent

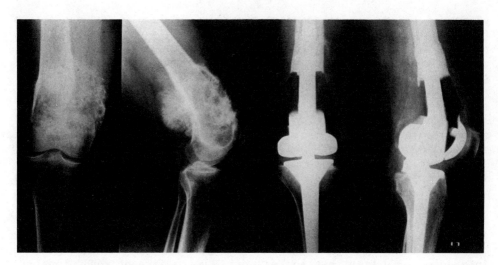

Fig. 3. Patient with fibroblastic grade II osteosarcoma of the
         distal femur. Local tumor resection performed with replace-
         ment by a custom made endoprosthesis. IFN therapy for 18
         months: six years later no evidence of disease, good
         function of the limb with full weight bearing and good walk-
         ing ability.

controls" and comprized all osteosarcoma patients in Sweden from 1972
onwards who were treated outside the Karolinska Hospital and
consequently did not receive IFN (Broström, 1979; Broström et al.,
1980; Strander et al., 1982). These concurrent controls, totalling
51 cases, consisted of a group of 30 patients who had received only
conventional treatment with irradiation and ablative surgery, and a
group of 21 patients treated during the latter part of the
observation period, who also received high-dose adjuvant treatment
with cytostatics.

     Since the three groups numerically are fairly small, their
comparability was checked by analysis of a number of prognostic
factors (Table I). Factors typical of primary classical osteosarcoma, such as age and sex distribution, symptomatology, tumor
type, size and localization, are held in common by all patients
(N=137). However, larger and more malignant tumors are found in the
historical control group. The incidence of osteoblastic Grade IV
tumors is about 80% in this group as compared to about 50% in the
other two groups. Except for the type of surgery performed, the IFN
group and the concurrent control group show good conformity with
respect to practically all the factors analyzed.

     At present the IFN group shows a five-year survival rate of 54%.
In the control group the five-year survival rate is 36% for concurrent controls and 14% for historical controls (Figs. 4 and 5). At
the five-year limit 44% of the patients in the IFN group are free of

TABLE I

Prognostic Factors

	Interferon		Concurrent controls Chemotherapy		Concurrent controls No adjuvant		Historical controls	
Males	32		13		18		22	
Females	19		8		12		13	
Age,yrs(mean±S.D.)	24	± 12	18 ±	5	16 ±	8	17 ±	9
Duration of symptoms prior to presentation,mo. (mean±S.D.)	4	± 5	3 ±	2	3,5 ±	2,5	3,5 ±	2,5
Size of tumor,cm (mean±S.D.)	10	± 3,5	10 ±	5	8,5 ±	3	13	± 6,5
Type of tumor:								
Osteoblastic	31	61%	11	52%	16	53%	29	83%
Chondroblastic	9	18%	5	24%	5	17%	4	12%
Fibroblastic	11	22%	5	24%	9	30%	2	6%
Grade of tumor:								
IV	26	51%	7	33%	17	57%	28	80%
III	19	37%	12	57%	11	37%	6	17%
II	6	12%	2	10%	2	5%	0	
Undefined	0		0		0		1	3%
Location of tumor:								
Proximal	29	57%	13	62%	18	60%	23	66%
Distal	22	43%	8	35%	12	40%	12	34%
Knee region	38	75%	14	67%	23	77%	25	71%
Type of tumor surgery:								
Disarticulation	6	12%	9	43%	7	23%	16	56%
Amputation	27	53%	12	57%	18	60%	14	40%
Local resection	17	33%	0		2	7%	0	
None	1	2%	0		3	10%	5	14%

metastases. In the control groups the corresponding rates are 33% for concurrent controls and 14% for historical controls (Fig. 3). The figures mentioned for the concurrent control group refer to the total survival and metastasis-free rates observed for both subgroups.

Osteosarcoma metastasizes predominantly to the lungs (Broström, 1979; Dahlin and Coventry, 1967). In the majority of patients

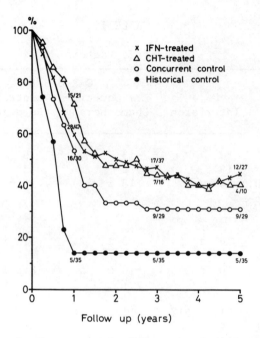

Fig. 4.   Metastasis free rate in IFN-treated patients.
          x———x (N=51) IFN-treated; △———△ chemotherapy treated
          (N=21); o———o no adjuvant therapy (N=30) and historical
          control group ●———● (N=35).

metastases are probably present already at the time of diagnosis in
microscopic form. Adjuvant therapy (IFN, chemotherapy) aims at
eliminating and possibly preventing such micrometastases. Prior to
1970, the treatment of known metastases was conservative. In recent
years various types of combined treatment (chemotherapy, irradiation)
have been attempted, with varying and often poor results. However,
in the IFN group eight patients have during the past few years been
treated with a combination of HuIFN-α and irradiation. IFN was
administered with a daily dosage of three million units, irradiation
of the lungs in a daily dose of 100-200 cGy with a maximum total
dosage of 2000 cGy. The treatment was tolerated well by all patients
and produced an improvement in general condition. In two cases
radiological regression of metastases could be noted. A longer
observation time of a larger series of patients is needed, however,
to permit any definite conclusions.

DISCUSSION

    The IFN group comprizes a consecutive series of patients with
classical osteosarcoma. No randomization of treatment was adopted in

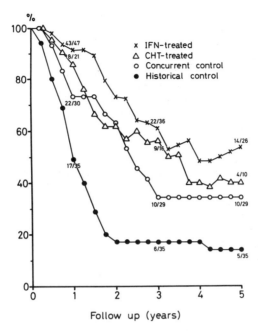

Fig. 5.   Survival rate in IFN-treated patients.
x——x (N=51) IFN-treated; △——△ chemotherapy treated
(N=21); o——o no adjuvant therapy (N=30) and historical
control group ●——● (N=35).

this clinical trial, since at the outset so-called historical
controls were believed to be a suitable instrument for comparison.
The poor prognosis for osteosarcoma at that time appeared to be so
well documented that any change in the course of the disease could be
interpreted as an effect of treatment.

Analysis of a number of prognostic factors, however, revealed
certain differences between the historical control group and the
interferon group (Broström et al., 1980). For example, the
historical control group showed a predominance of tumors presenting
histological criteria of high-grade malignancy. The interferon group
showed a lower incidence of tumors of this type (Table I). This
unexpected finding led to the addition of a group of concurrent
controls, comprizing all osteosarcoma patients treated in Sweden
without IFN adjuvance during the same observation period as the IFN
group. This second control group presented a similar difference in
comparison to the historical control group, consisting in a lower
incidence of cases of high-grade histologic malignancy. Variations
in incidences are known in oncology but the causes of such variations
are unknown. It is likewise unknown whether there may be shifts in
the natural history of a specific malignant tumor but at least in the

series included in our study there is an apparent verging towards a
more lenient clinical course (Broström, 1979). In this context it
may also be mentioned that the Mayo Clinic has reported a similar
increase in recent years in the survival rate for osteosarcoma
patients treated by surgery only (Taylor et al., 1978). It should be
emphasized, therefore, that historical control groups should be used
with critical discernment in clinical studies of malignant disease
and that any pertinent comparisons of the results of treatment demand
a long-term perspective.

Nevertheless, the IFN treated osteosarcoma series shows an
increased survival rate not only in comparison with the historical
control group, but also when compared with the concurrent controls.
So far the number of patients is not large enough to yield
statistically significant results, but at the clinical level this
form of adjuvant treatment for osteosarcoma obviously seems to affect
the natural course of the disease. The other alternative currently
used for adjuvant treatment of osteosarcoma is presented by cytotoxic
drugs (high-dose methotrexate, adriamycin, etc.). Without
elaborating the subject it may be noted that the results of IFN
treatment in osteosarcoma as measured in terms of five-year survival
are better than those reported for most series treated by cytotoxic
drugs (Cancer Treatment Reports, 1978; Cancer Treatment Reports,
1981). Another point to be taken into account here is that IFN
treatment has not produced any major side effects and in no case has
had to be discontinued because of adverse reactions, whereas
treatment by other drugs is associated with almost invariably severe,
and sometimes critical, side effects. So far there is no possibility
of comparing our IFN series with other series of osteosarcoma
patients subjected to this treatment, since only a few reports
describing small series of this kind have been published.

As yet we cannot specify the optimal conditions for interferon
treatment of osteosarcoma patients, but in its present form this
adjuvant therapy yields a survival rate of 55% at the five-year
follow-up. Metastases have developed in half of these cases, but an
increased supply of IFN of different types will open new possibilities of long-term and high-dose treatment. Experimental studies
have demonstrated synergistic antitumor effects produced on osteosarcoma by IFN-α and IFN-γ a combination which as yet has not been
clinically tested. Additional clinical and experimental studies are
needed to provide a clearer picture of the interaction both between
different types of IFN, and when combined with other forms of
antitumor therapy.

Our confidence in the positive effects of interferon in the
treatment of osteosarcoma has also led us to some extent to abandon
ablative surgery in favor of local tumor resection. The fact that
such local removal was performed in no less than 33% of the cases in
our IFN group makes it wholly unique in relation to all other

osteosarcoma series so far reported (Nilsonne and Strander, 1981).
The increased five-year survival rate in the IFN group would also
seem to justify our policy of performing local rather than ablative
surgery whenever possible.

REFERENCES

Balkwill, F., Taylor-Papadimitriou, J., Fantes, K., and Sebesteny, A.
1980, Human lymphoblastoid interferon can inhibit the growth of
human breast cancer xenografts in athymic (nude) mice. Europ.
J. Cancer, 16:569.
Balkwill, F. 1979, Interferons as cell-regulatory molecules. Cancer
Immunol. Immunother., 7:7.
Broström, L.-A. 1979, On the natural history of osteosarcoma.
Aspects on diagnosis, prognosis and endocrinology. Doctor's
thesis. Acta Orthop. Scand. Suppl., 183.
Broström, L.-A., Aparisi, T., Ingimarsson, S., Lagergren, C.,
Nilsonne, U., Strander, H., and Söderberg, G. 1980, Can
historical controls be used in current clinical trials in
osteosarcoma? Analysis of prognostic factors in a historical
and a contemporary group. Int. J. Rad. Oncol. Biol. Phys.,
6:1711.
Broström, L.-A. 1980, The combined effect of interferon and
methotrexate on human osteosarcoma and lymphoma cell lines.
Cancer Letters, 10:83.
Cancer Treatment Reports 1978, Proceedings of Osteosarcoma Study
Group Meeting Febr. 1978. National Cancer Inst. (NIH), USA.
Cancer Treat. Rep., 62:187.
Cancer Treatment Reports 1981, Proceedings of the International
Symposium on Methotrexate. National Cancer Inst. (NIH) USA.
Cancer Treat. Rep., 65 Suppl. 1:99.
Chirigos, M., and Pearson, J. 1973, Cure of murine leukaemia with
drug and interferon treatment. J. Natl. Cancer Inst., 51:1367.
Crane, J., Glasgow, L., Kern, E., and Younger, J. 1978, Inhibition of
murine osteogenic sarcomas by treatment with type I or type II
interferon. J. Natl. Cancer Inst., 61:871.
Dahlin, D., and Coventry, M. 1967, Osteogenic sarcoma: A study of six
hundred cases. J. Bone Jt. Surg., 45-A:101.
De Clercq, E., Georgiades, J., Edy, V., and Sobis, H. 1978, Effect of
human and mouse interferon and of polyriboinosinic acid, polyribocytidylic acid on the growth of human fibrosarcoma and
melanoma tumors in nude mice. Europ. J. Cancer, 14:1273.
Einhorn, S., and Strander, H. 1977, Is interferon tissue specific?
Effect of human leukocyte and fibroblast interferons on the
growth of lymphoblastoid and osteosarcoma cell lines. J. Gen.
Virol., 35:573.
Glasgow, L., Crane, J., Jr., and Kern, E. 1978, Antitumor activity of
interferon against murine osteogenic sarcoma cells in vitro. J.
Natl. Cancer Inst., 60:659.

Glasgow, L., and Kern, E. 1981, Effect of interferon administration
    on pulmonary osteogenic sarcomas in an experimental murine
    model. J. Natl. Cancer Inst., 67:207.
Glasgow, L., Crane, J., Schleupner, Ch., Kern, E., Younger, J., and
    Feingold, D. 1979, Enhancement of resistance to murine
    osteogenic sarcoma in vivo by an extract of Brucella abortus
    (Bur-Pel). Infect. and Immun., 23:1.
Gresser, I. 1977, Antitumor effects of interferon in: "Cancer - A
    Comprehensive Treatise (Chemotherapy)" 5:525, Plenum Publ.
    Corp., New York.
Gresser, I., Maury, C., and Tovey, M. 1978, Efficacy of combined
    interferon cyclophosphamide therapy after diagnosis of lymphoma
    in AKR mice. Eur. J. Cancer, 14:97.
Ingimarsson, S., Cantell, K., and Strander, H. 1979, Side effects of
    long-term treatment with human leukocyte interferon. J. Inf.
    Dis., 140:560.
Nilsonne, U., and Strander, H. 1981, Traitement de l'ostéosarcome par
    l'interféron et la chirurgie différenciée. Rev. Chir. Orthop.,
    67:193.
Paucker, K., Cantell, K., and Henle, W. 1962, Quantitative studies on
    viral interference in suspended L cells. III. Effect of
    interfering viruses and interferon on the growth rate of cells.
    Virology, 17:324.
Strander, H., and Einhorn, S. 1977, Effect of human leukocyte
    interferon on the growth of human osteosarcoma cells in tissue
    culture. Int. J. Cancer, 19:468.
Strander, H., Aparisi, T., Blomgren, H., Broström, L.-A., Cantell,
    K., Einhorn, S., Ingimarsson, S., Nilsonne, U., and Söderberg,
    G. 1982, Adjuvant interferon treatment of human osteosarcoma in:
    "Recent Results in Cancer Research 80", Springer Verlag, Berlin.
Taylor, W., Ivins, J., Dahlin, D., Edmonson, J., and Pritchard, D.
    1978, Trends and variability in survival from osteosarcoma, Mayo
    Clin. Proc., 53:695.

PAPILLOMAS

GEOFFREY M. SCOTT

Clinical Research Centre, Watford Road, Harrow, Middlesex

INTRODUCTION

This review will discuss the biology of the benign epithelial
tumors of man caused by papillomaviruses and the use of interferon in
their treatment. Although the effects of interferon on the replication of polyomaviruses, particularly Simian virus 40, in vitro have
been studied in detail (for review, see Stewart II, 1979), it is not
possible to extrapolate these data with justification to the replication of papillomaviruses which have proved rather tedious to grow
and pass in tissue culture. However, the study of the effects of
interferon against warts is of considerable interest because these
are the only tumors in man for which a viral etiology is not
disputed.

THE DISEASES

Warts are common transmissible benign tumors of skin and mucous
membranes (Bunney, 1975; Sanders and Stretcher, 1976; Haber et al.,
1980; Coleman, 1980). They may be classified according to their
anatomical sites and macroscopic appearances. Recent studies of the
papillomaviruses isolated from different types of warts lend credence
to the suggestion that simple clinical and pathological differences
do reflect different virus infections (Almeida et al., 1969). Warts
at any site may become malignant after many years.

Common warts (verruca vulgaris) may occur at any age but this is
primarily a disease of pre-adolescence or of certain occupations.
Warts are usually multiple and may occur anywhere although sites
prone to mild trauma such as the hand or the sole of the foot are

favored. Butchers (Ostrow et al., 1981; Orth et al., 1981) and
poultry workers (Taylor, 1980) develop warts on their hands. The
lesions are firm rough papules not often larger than 2 cm in diameter
but on the sole of the foot they may coalesce. Histologically, all
types of warts are characterized by hyperkeratosis and acanthosis
(Haber et al., 1980; Massing and Epstein, 1963). Proliferating cells
from the granular layer are thrown up into folds. There are atypical
vacuolated epidermal cells with eosinophilic nuclear and cytoplasmic
inclusions; the viral inclusions on the other hand, are basophilic
and restricted to the nucleus. Virus is shed in profusion with the
outer cell layers and is transmitted by direct contact, via surfaces
such as in swimming pools or via certain fomites (such as the glue
used in a cardboard box factory; McLaughlin and Edington, 1937) and
satellite lesions are common.

Plane warts (verrucae planae) have many of the characteristics
of simple body warts but are, as their name implies, flat papules
commonly distributed on exposed areas of the skin such as the backs
of the hands. An unusual condition of multiple planar warts, epidermodysplasia verruciformis (Lutzner, 1978), is considered to be
familial, transmitted by an autosomal recessive gene. However, as
virus is found in these warts (Pfister et al., 1981), maybe it is
that susceptibility to infection or this particular manifestation is
inherited or that family contact is important in the spread of a
particular virus. Acanthosis and hyperkeratosis of the epidermis
with vacuolation of the cells is also seen in plane warts but the
disease does not appear histologically to be as exuberant as body
warts.

Genital warts (condylomata acuminata: Oriel, 1971a,b) appear in
the anogenital regions. This disease is quite different from body
warts. It is acquired at sexual maturity and virus is probably
transmitted by sexual contact. Warts are grouped around muco-
cutaneous junctions and although epidermal changes are histologically
similar to body warts, the lesions themselves are soft, bulky and
often almost pedunculated. They are oedematous and infiltrated by
inflammatory cells. They may become very large particularly in
pregnancy or during immunosuppression. Although it used to be
thought that genital warts were a manifestation of gonorrhoea and
more recently that they were body warts modified by the environment
in which they were growing, recent studies have demonstrated that at
least one different species of papillomavirus is involved.

Juvenile laryngeal papilloma is a rare condition of very young
children (Ullman, 1923; Cohen et al., 1980; Anonymous, 1981).
Multiple small warty growths are distributed over the mucosa of the
larynx sometimes extending into the pharynx and down into the
tracheobronchial tree and lung parenchyma. They grow and coalesce,
causing stridor and respiratory obstruction. Histologically, they
are similar to genital warts with proliferation of the stratified

squamous epithelium and multiple papillary processes thrown up from the granular layer (Friemann and Osborne, 1976). Because they are mobile and not keratinized, they are more like genital warts than body warts and it has been proposed that infection is acquired from the birth canal during parturition (Cook et al., 1973; Quick et al., 1980). However, Ullman (1923) observed that body warts were more common in children with juvenile laryngeal papillomas than those without, suggesting an altered susceptibility to infection. In adults, this condition is exceedingly rare but isolated firm papillomas on the larynx may occur; these have on occasion been shown to contain papillomavirus (Boyle et al., 1973). Adults may also rarely develop an unpleasant florid oral papillomatosis with multiple warty growths on the buccal surfaces but this is quite unlike juvenile laryngeal papillomas and may be an unusual manifestation of body warts or genital warts.

NATURAL HISTORY

Spontaneous Resolution

Warts are benign tumors but they tend to persist for months or years before resolving spontaneously (Massing and Epstein, 1963). The mechanism for this is not clear. Circulating antibodies to wart virus were detected by electron microscopy and immunodiffusion but there was no difference in the presence of these antibodies before and after treatment (Almeida and Goffe, 1965). More recently, Pyrhönen and Johansson (1975) found that patients with warts who had detectable circulating IgG antibodies which fixed complement (about 20% of a population of 173), had a more rapid response to standard treatment than those with IgM antibodies detectable by immuno-diffusion. However, the presence of antibodies is not directly associated with spontaneous resolution of warts, and the failure of active immunization by autogenous vaccination (Biberstein, 1944) suggests that cell-mediated responses are involved (Allison, 1966). Moreover, warts proliferate in conditions of depressed cell-mediated immunity (Spencer and Andersen, 1970; Morison, 1974a).

Biberstein (1944) showed autogenous vaccination with wart tissues to cause inflammation around the bases of warts away from the vaccination site. About a month before multiple planar warts of epidermodysplasia verruciformis resolve spontaneously, there is a marked inflammation around the base of these warts (Tagami et al., 1980); histologically a massive mononuclear cell infiltrate but no specific deposits of immunoglobulins or complement are seen. Oguchi et al. (1981) used ultrastructural studies to demonstrate activation of macrophages against infected cells. Genetic differences in immune responses to papillomaviruses are illustrated by the observation that Shope rabbit papillomavirus (Shope, 1933) can be passaged repeatedly in the natural host, the cottontail rabbit, but not in domestic rabbits which generate a good neutralizing antibody response.

Morison (1974b) found an increase in cell-mediated reponse to wart antigen as measured by leukocyte migration inhibition tests before and after treatment. Resistant warts have been treated by applying dinitrochlorobenzene (DNCB) to the lesions in previously sensitized patients. This would be expected to induce a local delayed hypersensitivity reaction (Greenberg et al., 1973; Petrelli et al., 1981). In one sensitized patient with multiple body warts which were refractory to conventional treatments, DNCB had no effect on the lesions themselves, although it induced a reaction in normal skin. A factor produced in the wart which could block local cell-mediated reactions was proposed (Freed and Eyres, 1979). A similar approach to DNCB was to try mumps skin test antigen given into the base of juvenile laryngeal papillomata in a child previously actively immunized against mumps (Grensher, 1980) . The papillomas resolved but recurred a few months later. Levamisole has also been tried with a degree of success in patients with multiple warts (Moncada and Rodriguez, 1979). These data provide indirect evidence that cell-mediated immune responses are important in the resolution of warts but the trigger for such an event in a patient who has had warts for year remains an enigma.

Malignant Change

All warts may progress to carcinoma-in-situ or frank invasive carcinoma after a latent period of many years. For epidermodysplasia verruciformis, this is not an uncommon event (Lutzner, 1978), but for laryngeal papillomas and condylomata acuminata it is rare (Siegel, 1962), and for verrucae, it is so rare as to warrant the very occasional case report (Goette, 1980). One of the 90 cases of laryngeal papillomas reviewed by Cohen et al. (1980), developed a bronchial carcinoma. This child had had over 100 operative procedures to remove papillomas, and repeated operations or radiation therapy are thought to be associated with an increased risk of malignant change. Although oncogenesis appears to be an important property of all the papovaviruses, when malignancy supervenes virus is not detectable in the cells of the tumor. A case can be made for papillomavirus as causing some common skin, vulval and cervical carcinomas (Zur Hausen, 1976; Bender and Pass, 1981; Rapp and Jenkins, 1981).

PAPILLOMAVIRUSES

Warts may be transmitted to healthy recipients by the intradermal inoculation of crude extracts, cell free extracts and ultrafiltered extracts of all types of human warts (Ullman, 1923; Goldschmidt and Kligman, 1958). The appearances of these experimental lesions in normal skin are similar, suggesting that they might be caused by the same virus. The first evidence that there is heterogeneity in the viruses was provided by Almeida et al. (1969)

who showed that antisera raised against genital warts virus did not
react with body wart virus.

Virus particles were seen by electron microscopy of extracts of
body warts (Strauss et al., 1949), genital warts (Oriel and Almeida,
1970) and laryngeal papillomas (Boyle et al., 1971). Virus particles
may be seen in the nuclei of ultrathin sections of body warts: the
number of particles per cell increases towards the outer layers of
the lesions (Almeida et al., 1962). Viruses are rarely seen in
sections from genital warts and juvenile laryngeal papillomata.

Papovaviruses (of which papillomaviruses form a subgroup of
particle size 50-55 nm, a little larger than polyomaviruses) are DNA
viruses with icosahedral symmetry. The DNA exists as a single
double-stranded ring and replicates in the cell nucleus (Melnick et
al., 1974; Andrewes et al., 1976). Human papillomaviruses are slow
to grow and difficult to pass in tissue culture (Rowson and Mahy,
1967; Quick et al., 1978) and this has hindered the study of their
biology.

Following the demonstration of different serotypes of papillomaviruses, more sensitive techniques using molecular hybridization
showed that one probe for the DNA from plantar warts can react with
DNA from body warts but not genital warts or juvenile laryngeal
papillomas (Zur Hausen et al., 1976; Delap et al., 1976). Favre et
al. (1975) mapped one human papillomavirus genome using restriction
endonucleases. A major difference in DNA sequence between a hand and
a plantar wart virus was shown by Orth et al. (1977) and Staquet et
al. (1979) also found quite different virus polypeptides in plantar
and hand warts. Two new viruses with no DNA sequence homology which
did not cross-react antigenically were isolated from different
patients with epidermodysplasia verruciformis. One was preferentially associated with malignant change (Orth et al., 1978). By
1980, the existence of five different human papillomaviruses (HPV)
had been agreed by different groups (Coleman, 1980). Since then,
Pfister et al. (1981) have been able to isolate a new HPV from one
patient with epidermodysplasia verruciformis and Ostrow et al. (1981)
and Orth et al. (1981) have both found new HPV's in the warts of meat
handlers. Boyle et al. (1971) indicated that only 10-20% of
laryngeal papillomas have demonstrable virus by electron microscopy
but a reaction between hyperimmune rabbit anti-bovine papillomavirus
I proteins and the cell nuclei of about half 102 human laryngeal
papillomas confirms the presence of papillomaviruses with common
antigenic determinants (Lack et al., 1980). Similarly three out of
four juvenile laryngeal papillomas had intranuclear antigen in the
differentiating granular layer identified by antibody against bovine
papillomavirus I (Lancaster and Jenson, 1981). Positive
hybridization could be demonstrated between HPV probes and both
laryngeal papillomas and condylomata providing convincing evidence
that the two are related (Quick et al., 1980).

It seems likely that different types of warts will prove to be associated with specific HPV's and that unusual manifestations of infections may arise because of infection with an uncommon virus for that site.

TREATMENT

There is an extraordinary range of treatments recommended for warts, ranging from folk remedies to sophisticated modern drugs and surgical techniques (Bunney, 1975). Whereas charming warts away does not appear to be very efficient (Clarke, 1965), all claims for a cure are aided by the spontaneous resolution of warts. Perhaps the most acceptable treatment for body or genital warts is the repeated application of liquid nitrogen or solid carbon dioxide. Surgery is reserved for those who fail to respond to this conservative treatment and currettage, diathermy or cryotherapy are preferable to excision which causes scarring. Various topical agents (caustics, formaldehyde, glutaraldehyde or salicylic acid) may be incorporated into proprietary preparations. No treatment guarantees cure with a single application and most have to be repeated for weeks or months (Bunney, 1975; Simmons, 1981; Simmons et al., 1981). Only 22% of 140 patients were free of genital warts after three months' weekly applications of podophylin (Simmons, 1981). Several other anti-metabolites such as fluorouracil (Smith et al., 1980), methotrexate (van der Beek et al., 1980) or bleomycin (Abbott, 1978) have been used with some success in resistant cases of florid oral papilloma-tosis, juvenile or verrucae.

Surgical removal or cautery via laryngoscopy is indicated for juvenile laryngeal papillomas but they recur with monotonous regularity and repeated procedures under general anaesthetic are usually required. Tracheotomy may also be needed but may predispose to lower respiratory tract seeding (Cohen et al., 1980). Intractable juvenile laryngeal papillomas have been successfully treated with Bleomycin (Mehta and Herold, 1980). Pritchard et al. (1980) have used adenine arabinoside in six children requiring frequent surgery. Three of the six responded with prolongation of the intervals between operations. Slightly better results were seen with topical fluoro-uracil and all of eight patients showed some improvement using the same criterion (Smith et al., 1980). Among the immune enhance- ment procedures mentioned above, levamisole (Schouten et al., 1981) and local mumps skin test antigen (Grensher, 1980) have been tried with limited success.

McGee (1967) used either virulent or partly heat-attenuated vaccinia virus to treat body virus warts at various sites. Attenuated virus was used on sensitive areas of skin but virulent virus was used against warts in areas naturally resistant to vaccination such as the palms. In 60 patients, 164/165 warts showed

varying degrees to local reaction after one or more vaccinations
(using multiple pressure technique) and then disappeared leaving no
scar. However, Allyn and Waldorf (1968) repeated this work in
smaller numbers of patients using virulent virus and found that there
was a considerable risk of morbidity. The response of the warts was
associated with the degree of inflammation seen. If there was no
reaction to vaccination, the wart did not change. However, McGee
(1967) also showed that warts did not resolve by causing local
inflammation with nitric acid or using various other killed vaccines
(including DPT and polio). Hutchinson (1970) used virulent vaccinia
virus in the warts in 100 patients. About one month after treatment,
the wart was necrotic and sharply delineated from the surrounding
tissue. If this necrotic wart was removed, the overall cure rate was
79%. It was proposed that vaccinia virus acted by viral interference, perhaps by inducing interferon. The technique has fallen
out of favour, either because of the morbidity involved or because of
a reluctance to use live vaccinia virus for a trivial condition now
that the threat of smallpox has gone. It seemed natural, however, to
try interferons not only because they have antiviral properties but
because of their cytostatic and immune-enhancement effects.

Interferon Therapy

     In Russia, patients with body or plantar warts were subjected to
various regimes of topical interferon ointment therapy (1000 u/g)
(Borzov et al., 1971). Local application of interferon alone seemed
ineffective so a method of traumatizing the skin by rubbing with a
toothbrush before applying the interferon was tried. Five out of
eight cases so treated had "a good result" which was not defined.

     Twenty-eight patients then had injections of crude leukocyte
interferon into body or plantar warts. This resulted in resolution
of all the warts in between seven and 20 days with no recurrences
over a two-year period. Similarly, repeated injections of interferons into genital warts appeared a successful treatment but the
number of cases treated was not clear from the report. The
concentration or dose of interferon was not given and none of
Borzov's studies appear to have been controlled.

     Ikić and coworkers in Yugoslavia have studied the effects of
interferon cream or ointment preparations on genital warts. The
preparations contained 4000 u freeze-dried crude leukocyte interferon
per gram of base, which was to be applied five times per day. In the
first uncontrolled study (Ikić et al., 1975a) forty women with vulval
warts treated themselves for between one and eight weeks. All but
four showed complete regression of the warts by eight weeks after
starting the treatment. In three, the treatment was discontinued at
five weeks and in one at eight weeks, no noticeable change having
been observed.

A double-blind controlled trial was then performed comparing the effects of the same preparation of interferon with placebo ointments in twenty women with vulval warts. All those in the interferon group showed complete regression but it took twelve weeks in three of them. Three out of ten patients on placebo showed regression of the warts at three, four and six weeks but three others showed progression (Ikić et al., 1975b). Five patients who had not responded to placebo treatment were then cured using the active preparation within an average period of eight weeks (Smerdel et al., 1976).

Finally, a further open study comparing the treatment of men with penile warts and women with vulval warts using either a cream or ointment formulation showed an overall response in one half of all the subjects (20/40) (Ikić et al., 1975c). In the successfully-treated group, the average time to regression of the warts was nine weeks. The response rate in men (14/32) differed from that in women (6/8). This suggested a difference in susceptibility of penile and vulval warts or a difference in compliance between men and women. No differences could be detected between effects of the interferon cream or ointment. Interferon ointment is now available from pharmacists in Yugoslavia and other Eastern bloc countries for the treatment of warts and herpesvirus infections. In 1977, a tube of 5 g (4000 u/g) was purchased by the author over the counter in Zagreb for about 10 US dollars but its activity was never established!

A small study was performed to assess the effect of injections of small doses of crude fibroblast interferon into penile warts (Scott and Csonka, 1979). The growth of the warts injected with interferon was compared with the growth of untreated warts and those injected with mock interferon. Perhaps only 300 u of fibroblast interferon were given in the active preparation and yet there was a significant reduction in wart growth compared with that of the controls. In one patient the wart injected with interferon disappeared within two weeks.

Ho and co-workers (1981) have studied in detail the effects of different dose schedules of partially purified leukocyte interferon in one patient with intractable multiple body warts which had been present for eight years. Despite the enhancement of circulating natural killer cell activity, parenteral interferon (2.4×10^6 u twice a week for 55 injections) had no effect on the skin lesions. On the other hand, local injections of interferon into the warts themselves did appear to have some effect. A total of 20×10^6 u given as 1.2×10^6 u intralesionally twice a week for seven weeks caused a decrease in the keratinization of one plantar wart (which was excised at the end of treatment) and resolution of one other, three weeks later. Different lesions injected with the same schedule of interferon disappeared at 16 weeks (treated for 14.5 weeks), nine weeks (treated for the whole period) and seven weeks (treated for five weeks). Interestingly, control lesions injected with placebo all showed some slight reduction in volume over the period of observation.

One case report of a patient whose plantar wart resolved while under treatment with partially purified leukocyte interferon parenterally for cervical carcinoma, was presented by Strander and Cantell (1974). This stimulated an open treatment trial of seven children with juvenile laryngeal papillomas at the Karolinska Institute, Stockholm between 1976 and 1980. They were given leukocyte interferon intramuscularly starting at 3×10^6 u three times a week and then reducing (Haglund et al., 1981). All the children required frequent surgery up to the time of treatment. Although complete details of the periods of treatment and the frequencies of surgery are not always given in the case summaries presented in this report, it is clear that there were no major recurrences of warts after surgical removal and no major progression of established disease on this schedule of interferon by one month after starting treatment. Large masses of tumor did not resolve spontaneously on treatment and it was considered essential to continue endoscopic surgery to remove all the warty tissue. Interferon was associated with a reduced frequency of surgery but in some cases, small warts persisted in the larynx despite interferon treatment. However, when treatment was stopped, the tumors recurred within two months. Seventeen full courses of interferon were started, ten after recurrences. If interferon was continued at a lower dose (2×10^6 u twice a week, or 10^6 u once a week) warts recurred but after four or five months. According to the report, therefore, several patients were continuing on regular interferon indefinitely in order to prevent recurrences.

Two other children were given 2×10^6 u fibroblast interferon intravenously daily for six weeks (Göbel et al., 1981). In one there was no progression of the disease, but in the other progression occurred requiring tracheotomy. After an interval, a change was made to subcutaneous leukocyte interferon at the same dose. After four weeks the tumors had regressed but a reduction in dose in one child to 10^6 u on alternate days was associated with a recurrence controlled by 2×10^6 u daily. In the other child, a reduction in dose to 2×10^6 u on alternate days did not control the disease but 10^6 u daily appeared to be satisfactory.

Two further children with extensive laryngeal papillomas extending into the lung parenchyma were treated with the synthetic double-stranded polyribonucleotide Poly ICLC, which is an efficient interferon inducer and immune adjuvant protected against circulating nucleases (Leventhal et al., 1981). In one boy there was a reduction in the requirement for surgical removal of warts during two courses of therapy given three times a week, and inducing serum levels of 20-800 u/ml interferon, eight hr after injection. Maintenance treatment once a week induced levels of 200-300 u/ml but repeated surgery continued to be necessary. Similar levels were induced in the second child and there was a modest reduction in the need for surgical interventions compared with a pre-trial period. There were

no changes in the radiological appearances of the disease in the
chest in either child and the treatment was associated with
considerable morbidity and hematologic toxicity. This was not unlike
the administration of some cytotoxic drugs, but more than reported
for bleomycin, which ine one case report, was considerably more
effective (Mehta and Herold, 1980).

DISCUSSION

From these preliminary trials, the effects of interferon on
warts can be summarized as follows. Local but not systemic leukocyte
interferon may induce the resolution of verrucae. On the other hand,
regular use of parenteral interferon appears to prevent recurrences
of juvenile laryngeal papillomas after surgical removal. Fibroblast
interferon may be less effective than leukocyte interferon but a
proper comparison has yet to be made. The dose of interferon and
length of treatment needed to induce resolution of verrucae has not
been established and the effects of very large doses given
systemically remain to be seen. The problems of material supply have
now been eased considerably by the insertion and expression of
interferon genes in bacteria or yeasts.

Interferons could work by inhibiting papillomavirus replication,
by suppressing the growth of proliferating epidermal cells, or by
enhancing cell-mediated immune responses to the tumor cells or virus.
It seems unlikely the latter is involved in the response of verrucae
to local interferon, because the effect on distal warts is minimal
when intralesional treatment is successful or when interferon is
given systemically. One further possibility is that intralesional
interferons work by inducing a non-specific inflammatory response and
that cellular recruitment into a lesion is sufficient to begin an
attack. We have shown that a monoclonal antibody-purified leukocyte
interferon preparation injected intradermally causes intense local
inflammation beginning at two - four hr, maximal around eight hr and
lasting more than 24 hr (Scott et al., 1981). However, leukocyte
interferon purified chemically (Scott et al., 1980) and IFNα2 from E.
coli (Schering Plough) did not appear to cause such reactions.
Whether the inflammation is caused by trace contaminants not removed
by monoclonal antibody separation or by subspecies of the alpha-
interferon family is not yet known. It should be possible to assess
the role of the inflammatory response in resolution of warts by
comparing different interferon preparations.

The difference in the type of response of juvenile papillomas
and verrucae may reflect a variable sensitivity of the different
papillomaviruses. This cannot be tested in vitro because of the slow
growth of these viruses in tissue culture. The behavior, appearance
and natural history of verrucae suggest that this is an anergic
condition when compared with juvenile laryngeal papillomas and

genital warts, in which virus is scarce and lesions have a mononuclear cell infiltrate. Laryngeal papillomas may be more
susceptible than verrucae to cell-mediated immune responses (for
example, NK cell or macrophage activation) enhanced by systemic
interferon. If this is so, then genital warts which are similar to
juvenile laryngeal papillomas should respond as well as the latter to
parenteral interferon. However, it is unlikely that repeated
injections of the sort of doses of interferon which appear to be
needed to affect laryngeal papillomas would be tolerated by patients
with this trivial illness which can be treated topically.
Furthermore, the response of laryngeal papillomas to interferon or
Poly ICLC has not been startling. If recurrences can be prevented
using a non-toxic dose, then interferon may have a role to play in
the routine therapy of this disease. It is suspicious that the doses
needed to prevent recurrences are just in the "toxic" range (Scott et
al., 1981) and that patients suffer fever and malaise. Perhaps
non-specific effects of parenteral interferon are important. Further
trials are necessary, preferably on a multi-centered basis,
appropriately controlled, comparing interferon with other standard
and novel therapies, such as adenine arabinoside, fluorouracil or
bleomycin. Perhaps a combination of interferon and adenine
arabinoside would be synergistic. Some way of quantifying the
results should be introduced to allow inter-trial comparisons. A
useful measure would be intervals between operations performed for
laryngeal obstruction.

The East European work on the topical use of crude interferon
preparations is of great interest. If it can be shown that intralesional interferon is effective against body or genital warts, then
topical preparations should be tested. The nature of the diseases
suggests that double-blind placebo-controlled or comparative trials
in large numbers of patients are essential to prove effects. If
topical interferon is effective against genital warts, then a simple
inhalational treatment could be tried in juvenile laryngeal
papillomas, particularly those invading the lung.

How far interferon treatment of warts should be pursued depends
not only on efficacy but also on its availability, its eventual price
and its lack of toxicity. Furthermore, it must be shown to have
clear advantages over present treatment methods.

REFERENCES

Abbott, L.G. 1978, Treatment of warts with bleomycin, Australas J.
    Dermatol., 19:69.
Allison, A.C. 1966, Immune responses to Shope fibromavirus in adult
    and newborn rabbits, J. Natl. Cancer Inst., 36:869.
Allyn, B. and Waldorf, D.S. 1968, Treatment of verruca with vaccinia,
    JAMA, 203:807.

Almeida, J.D. and Goffe, A.P. 1965, Antibody to wart virus in human
    sera demonstrated by electron microscopy and precipitin tests,
    Lancet, ii:1205.
Almeida, J.D., Howatson, A.F. and Williams, M.G. 1962, Electron
    microscope study of human warts, J. Invest. Dermatol., 38:337.
Almeida, J.D., Oriel, J.D. and Stannard, L.M. 1969, Characterisation
    of the virus found in human genital warts, Microbios., 1:225.
Andrewes, C.H., Perreira, H.G. and Wildy, P. 1976, Papovaviridae in:
    "Viruses of Vertebrates," p.273, Baillière-Tindall-London.
Anonymous. 1981, Multiple papillomas of the larynx in children,
    Lancet, i:367.
Bender, M.E. and Pass, F. 1981, Papillomavirus and cutaneous
    malignancy, Int. J. Dermatol., 20:468.
Biberstein, H. 1944, Immunization therapy of warts, Archives of
    Dermtatology and Syphilogy, 50:12.
Borzov, M.V., Kuznetsov, V.P. and Lobanovski, I. 1971, Relating to
    the use of interferon for the treatment and prevention of viral
    dermatoses, Vestnik dermatologii i venereologii, 45:14.
Boyle, W.F., McCoy, E.G. and Fogarty, F.W. 1971, Electron microscopic
    identification of virus-like particles in laryngeal papillomas,
    Ann. Otol., 80:693.
Boyle, W.F., Riggs, J.L., Oshiro, J.S. and Lennette, E.G. 1973,
    Electron microscopic identification of papoviruses in laryngeal
    papilloma, Laryngoscope, 83:1102.
Bunney, M.H. 1975, Warts, Hospital Medicine, 13:565.
Clarke, G.H. 1965, The charming of warts, J. Invest. Dermatol.,
    45:15.
Cohen, S.R., Geller, K.A., Seltzer, S. and Thompson, J.W. 1980,
    Papilloma of the larynx and tracheobronchial tree in children,
    Ann. Otol., 89:497.
Coleman, D.V. 1980, Recent developments in the papovaviruses: The
    human papillomaviruses in: "Recent Advances in Clinical
    Virology", Vol.2, p.79, A.P. Waterson, ed., Churchill
    Livingstone, Edinburgh.
Cook, J.A., Cohn, A.M., Brunschwig, J.P., Butel, J.S. and Rawls, W.E.
    1973, Wart virus and laryngeal papillomas, Lancet, i:782.
Delap, R., Friedman-Kien, A. and Rush, M.G. 1976, The absence of
    human papilloma viral DNA sequences in condyloma acuminata,
    Virology, 74:268.
Favre, M., Orth, G., Croissant, O. and Yaniv, M. 1975, Human
    papilloma virus DNA: physical map, Proc. Natl. Acad. USA,
    72:4810.
Freed, D.L. and Eyres, K.E. 1979, Persistent warts protected from
    immune attack by a blocking factor, Br. J. Dermatol., 100:731.
Friedmann, I. and Osborne, D.A. 1976, The larynx in: "Systemic
    Pathology", Vol.1, p.256, W. StC. Symmers, ed., Churchill
    Livingstone, Edinburgh.
Gobel, V., Arnold, W., Wahn, V., Treuner, J., Jurgens, H. and
    Cantell, K. 1981, Comparison of human fibroblast and leukocyte
    interferon in the treatment of severe laryngeal papillomatosis
    in children, Eur. J. Pediatr., 137:175.

Goette, K. 1980, Carcinoma in situ in verruca vulgaris, Int. J. Dermatol., 19:98.

Goldschmidt, H. and Kligman, A.M. 1958, Experimental inoculation of humans with ectodermic viruses, J. Invest. Dermatol., 31:175.

Greenberg, J.G., Smith, L. and Katz, R.M. 1973, Verrucae Vulgaris Rejection, Arch. Dermatol., 107:580.

Grensher, A. 1980, Treatment of laryngeal papillomas with mumps skin test antigens, Lancet, ii:920.

Haber, H., Milne, J.A. and Symmers, W.StC. 1980, in: "Systemic Pathology", Vol.6, p.2720, W. StC., Symmers, ed., Churchill Livingstone, Edinburgh.

Haglund, S., Lundquist, P.G., Cantell, K. and Strander, H. 1981, Interferon therapy in juvenile laryngeal papillomatosis, Arch. Otolaryngol., 107:327.

Ho, M., Pazin, G.J., White, L.T., Haverkos, H., Wechsler, R.L., Breinig, M.K., Cantell, K. and Armstrong, J.A. 1981, Intralesional treatment of warts with interferon-α and its long term effect on NK cell activity in: "The Biology of the Interferon System", p.361, E. DeMaeyer, G. Gallasso & H. Schellekens, eds., Elsevier, North Holland.

Hutchinson, R. 1970, The treatment of warts by viral interference, Practitioner, 204:700.

Ikić, D., Orescanin, M., Krusić, J., Cestar, Z., Alac, Z., Soos, E., Jusić, D. and Smerdel, S. 1975a, Preliminary study of the effect of human leukocytic interferon on condyolomata acuminata in women, in:"Proc. Symposium on Clinical Use of Interferon", p.223, D. Iki´, ed., Yugoslav Academy of Sciences and Arts, Zagreb.

Ikić, D., Bosnić, N., Smerdel, S., Jusić, D., Soos, E. and Delimar, N. 1975b, Double blind study with human leukocyte interferon in the therapy of condyolomata acuminata, in: "Proc. Symposium on Clinical Use of Interferon", p.229, D. Ikić, ed., Yugoslav Academy of Sciences and Arts, Zagreb.

Ikić, D., Brnobić, A., Jurković-Vukelić, V., Smerdel, S., Jusić, D., and Soos, E. 1975c, Therapeutical effect of human leukocyte interferon incorporated into ointment and cream on condyolomata acuminata, in: "Proc. Symposium on Clinical Use of Interferon", p.235, D. Ikić, ed., Yugoslav Academy of Sciences and Arts, Zagreb.

Lack, E.D., Vawter, G.F., Smith, H.G., Healy, G.B., Lancaster, W.D. and Jenson, A.B. 1980, Immunochemical localization of human papillomavirus in squamous papillomas of the larynx, Lancet, ii:592.

Lancaster, W.D. and Jenson, A.B. 1981, Evidence for papillomavirus genus-specific antigens and DNA in laryngeal papilloma, Intravirology, 15:204.

Leventhal, B.G., Kashima, H., Levine, A.S. and Levy, H.B. 1981, Treatment of recurrent laryngeal papillomatosis with an artificial interferon inducer, (Poly ICLC), J. Pediatrics, 99:614.

Lutzner, M.A. 1978, Epidermodysplasia verruciformis. An autosomal
     recessive disease characterized by viral warts and skin cancer.
     A model for viral oncogenesis, Bull Cancer (Paris), 65:169.
McGee, A.R. 1967, Wart treatment by vaccination with smallpox
     vaccine: a preliminary report, Canad. Med. Ass. J., 99:119.
McLaughlin, A.I.G. and Edington, J.W. 1937, Infective warts and bone
     glue, Lancet, ii:685.
Massing, A.M. and Epstein, W.L. 1963, Natural history of warts: a two
     year study, Arch. Dermatol., 87:306.
Mehta, P. and Herold, N. 1980, Regression of juvenile
     laryngobronchial papillomatosis with systemic bleomycin therapy,
     J. Pediatrics, 97:479.
Melnick, J.L., Allison, A.C. and Butel, J.S. 1974, Papovaviridae,
     Intervirology, 3:106.
Moncada, B. and Rodriguez, M.L. 1979, Levamisole therapy for multiple
     warts, Br. J. Dermatol., 101:327.
Morison, W.L. 1974a, Survey of viral warts, herpes zoster and herpes
     simplex in patients with secondary immune deficiencies and
     neoplasms, Br. J. Dermatol., 91:18.
Morison, W.L. 1974b, In vitro assay of cell-mediated immunity to
     human wart antigen, Br. J. Dermatol., 90:531.
Oguchi, M., Komura, J., Tagami, H. and Ofuji, S. 1981,
     Ultrastructural studies of spontaneously regressing plane warts.
     Macrophage attack verruca-epidermal cells, Arch. Dermatol. Res.,
     270:403.
Oriel, J.D. 1971a, Natural history of genital warts, Br. J. Vener.
     Dis., 47:1.
Oriel, J.D. 1971b, Anal warts and anal coitus, Br. J. Vener. Dis.,
     47:373.
Oriel, J.D. and Almeida, J.D. 1970, Demonstration of virus particles
     in human genital warts, Br. J. Vener. Dis., 46:37.
Orth, G., Favre, M. and Croissant, O. 1977, Characterisation of a new
     type of human papillomavirus that causes skin warts, J.
     Virology, 24:108.
Orth, G., Jablonska, S., Favre, M., Croissant, O.,
     Jarzabek-Chorzelska, M. and Rzesa, G. 1978, Characterization of
     two types of human papillomaviruses in lesions of
     epidermodysplasia verruciformis, Proc. Natl. Acad. Sci. USA,
     75:1537.
Orth, G., Jablonska, S., Favre, M., Croissant, O., Obalek, S.,
     Jarzabek-Chorzelsa, M. and Jibard, N. 1981, Identification of
     papillomavirus in butcher's warts, J. Invest. Dermatol., 76:97.
Ostrow, R.S., Krzyzek, R., Pass, F. and Faras, A.J. 1981,
     Identification of a novel human papillomavirus in cutaneous
     warts of meat handlers, Virology, 108:21.
Petrelli, R., Cotlier, E., Robins, S. and Stoessel, K. 1981,
     Dinitrochlorobenzene immunotherapy of recurrent squamous
     papilloma of the conjunctiva, Ophthalmology (Rochester),
     88:1221.

Pfister, H., Nürnberger, F., Gissmann, L. and Zur Hausen, H. 1981, Characterization of a human paillomavirus from epidermodysplasia verruciformis lesions of a patient from Upper Volta, Int. J. Cancer, 27:645.

Pritchard, J., Marshall, W.C., Eggerding, C., Pracy, R., Evans, J.N., Tymm, G., Innes, A. and Singh, A. 1980, Treatment of laryngeal papillomatosis, Lancet, ii:1383.

Pyrhönen, S. and Johansson, E. 1975, Regression of warts: an immunological study, Lancet, i:592.

Quick, C.A., Faras, A., and Krzysek, R. 1978, The aetiology of laryngeal papillomatosis, Laryngoscope, 88:1789.

Quick, C.A., Watts, S.L., Krzysek, R.A. and Faras, A.J. 1980, Relationship between condylomata and laryngeal papillomata. Clinical and molecular virological evidence, Ann. Otol., 89:467.

Rapp, F. and Jenkins, F.J. 1981, Genital cancer and viruses, Gynecol. Oncol., 12:S25.

Rowson, K.E. and Mahy, B.W. 1967, Human papova (wart) virus, Bacteriol. Rev,, 31:110.

Sanders, B.B. and Stretcher, G.S. 1976, Warts, diagnosis and treatment, JAMA, 235:2859.

Schouten, T.J., Bos, J.H., Bos, C.F., van der Pot, P.J. and van den Broek, P. 1981, Levamisole in the treatment of juvenile laryngeal papillomataosis, Int. J. Pediatr. Oto Rhinolaryngol., 3:365.

Scott, G.M. and Csonka, G.W. 1979, Effect of injections of small doses of human fibroblast interferon into genital warts: a pilot study, Br. J. Vener Dis., 55:442.

Scott, G.M., Secher, D.S., Flowers, D., Bate, J., Cantell, K. and Tyrrell, D.A.J. 1981, Toxicity of interferon, Br. Med. J., 282:1345.

Scott, G.M., Stewart, W.E. II, Tyrrell, D.A.J., Cantell, K., Cartwright, T. and Edy, V.G. 1980, Skin reactions to interferon inoculations are reduced but not abolished by purification, J. Interferon Research, 1:79.

Shope, R.E. 1933, Infectious papillomatosis of rabbits, J. Exp. Med., 58:607.

Siegel, A. 1962, Malignant transformation of condyloma acuminatum. Review of the literature and report of a case, Am. J. Surg., 103:613.

Simmons, P.D. 1981, Podophyllin 10% and 25% in the treatment of anogenital warts. A comparative double-blind study, Br. J. Vener Dis., 57:208.

Simmons, P.D., Langlet, F. and Thin, R.N. 1981, Cryotherapy versus electrocautery in the treatment of genital warts, Br. J. Vener Dis., 57:273.

Smerdel, S., Bosnić, N., Soos, E., Delimar, N. and Ikić, D. 1976, Treatment of condylomata acuminata with human leucocyte interferon, Period Biol. 78, Suppl. 1:150.

Smith, H.G., Healy, G.B., Vaughan, C.W. and Strong, M.S. 1980, Topical chemotherapy of recurrent respiratory papillomatosis (a preliminary report), Ann. Otol., 89:472.

Spencer, E.S. and Andersen, H.K. 1970, Clinical evident non-terminal infections with herpesviruses and the wart virus in immunosuppressed renal allograft recipients, Br. Med. J., 1:251.

Staquet, M.J., Viac, J. and Thivolet, J. 1979, Antigenic relationships between polypeptides derived from plantar and hand wart viruses, J. Gen. Virol., 43:713.

Stewart, W.E. II. 1979, "The Interferon System", Springer Verlag, Wien-New York.

Strander, H. and Cantell, K. 1974, Studies on the antiviral and antitumour effects of human leukocyte interferon in vitro and in vivo in: "The Production and Use of Interferon for the Treatment and Prevention of Human Virus Infections", p.49, Tissue Culture Association, Rockville Md.

Strauss, M.J., Shaw, E.W., Bunting, H. and Melnick, J.L. 1949, Crystalline virus-like particles from skin papillomas characterized by intranuclear inclusion bodies, Proc. Soc. Expl. Biol. Med., 72:46.

Tagami, H., Oguchi, M. and Ofuji, S. 1980, The phenomenon of spontaneous regression of numerous flat warts: immunohistological studies, Cancer, 45:2557.

Taylor, S.W. 1980, A prevalence study of virus warts on the hands in a poultry-packing station, J. Soc. Occup. Med., 30:20.

Ullman, E.V. 1923, On the aetiology of laryngeal papilloma, Acta. Otolaryngol, 5:317.

van der Beek, J.M., Cremers, C.W. and van den Broek, P. 1980, Successful methotrexate therapy in oral florid papillomatosis, Clin. Otolaryngol, 5:365.

Zur Hausen, H. 1976, Condyloma acuminata and human genital cancer, Cancer Res., 36:794.

INTRALESIONAL THERAPY

DRAGO IKIĆ

Center for Research and Standardization of Immunologic
Substances, Department of Medical Sciences, Yugoslav
Academy of Sciences and Arts, Zagreb, Yugoslavia

Intralesional, perilesional and topical use of interferon have
advantages when compared to parenteral administration. Only a small
amount of active substance is required to reach the desired local
concentration. The effects of therapy can be assessed more easily
and the incidence of side effects is lower. We first used topical
human leukocyte interferon (HLI) in three patients in 1972. The
first patient developed recurrent carcinoma of the vulva following
vulvectomy, irradiation and chemotherapy (Ikić et al., 1975). The
vulval recurrence was 3 cm in diameter and was ulcerated. After
three weeks of therapy the tumor regressed. The patient, however,
had metastases in the inguinal lymph nodes. The patient lived for
one year. Death was caused by generalized metastases. The second
patient had a basal cell carcinoma. After daily intralesional
application of HLI for 30 days the site of the carcinoma was barely
visible on the skin. Subsequent biopsy revealed granuloma only. A
further patient with cervical carcinoma was given intralesional
treatment with HLI for 21 days followed by radical surgery (Ikić et
al., 1975). The histological findings after therapy were of
inflammatory changes only although before the application of HLI
invasive carcinoma had been histologically verified.

Over the last decade we have extended our studies on the effects
of local interferon administration to carcinoma of the cervix, head
and neck tumors, bladder papillomatosis and breast cancer. This
chapter reviews our results to date.

CARCINOMA OF THE UTERINE CERVIX

Carcinoma in Situ

We have investigated the effects of topical application of HLI
in patients with cervical intraepithelial neoplasia (CIN) grades

169

I-III in a randomized study. In the first group of patients crude
freeze-dried HLI was applied in the vagina topically in the form of
powder by means of an "Ortho" contraceptive pessary, at a daily dose
of 1 x 10^6 units. Therapy was continued for 21 days. Two patients
were excluded from the further follow-up because cone biopsies were
performed. The second group consisted of 18 patients with the same
histological findings. These patients were given placebo (lyophilized medium used for the preparation of HLI). The results of
this study over a period of two years are presented in Table I.

Cytological and histological findings in this randomized study
showed significant differences between the treated and the control
groups. In the control group the abnormal epithelium was persistent
in seven cases and there were seven progressions. No regressions
were recorded. In the HLI-treated group we found four cases of
persistent disease, one case of progression and eight cases with
regression of the malignant process. We conclude that HLI has an
impact on the regression of the cervical intraepithelial neoplasia,
and that therapy with HLI may be indicated in women in the
reproductive age in whom fertility is to be preserved, as surgery can
be avoided (Ikić et al., 1981a,b,c and d).

Invasive Carcinoma

Our investigations on the influence of HLI on invasive cervical
carcinoma began in 1972 and can be divided into three phases. In

TABLE I

Follow-up Results of HLI-Treated Patients
and Untreated Controls with CIS

Therapy	Findings before therapy	No.	Findings after two years				
			NC	CIN I/II	CIN III	CIS	CIM
Placebo	CIN I/II	14	0	7	0	5	2
	CIN III	4	0	0	0	4	0
	Total	18	0	7	0	9	2
HLI	CIN I/II	10	7	3	0	0	0
	CIN III	3	0	1	1	1	0
	Total	13	7	4	1	1	0

NC	Normal cells only
CIN I/II	Borderline lesions - cervical intraepithelial neoplasia
CIN III	Marked lesions - cervical intraepithelial neoplasia
CIS	Carcinoma in situ
CIM	Micro invasive carcinoma

phase one, the influence of HLI on cervical cancer administered by injection directly into the tumor was examined in ten patients (Ikić et al., 1975). The encouraging cytological and histological changes and the results of in vitro experiments prompted us to apply HLI topically in pessaries in 12 patients (Krusić et al., 1977). The histological findings in the stroma of the tumors and in the regional lymph nodes as well as the patients' tolerance of HLI encouraged us to proceed to the third phase – combined topical application and intramuscular injection.

Patients and Methods

15 patients aged 23 to 55 years (mean 41) with cervical carcinoma took part in the study.

Biopsies for histological and histochemical assessment were removed prior to HLI treatment; after 14 days treatment; and at the end of treatment. On completion of HLI therapy the patients were treated with surgery or radiation, depending on the histological findings in the primary tumor and in the regional lymph nodes.

In six patients HLI was applied only topically at 2×10^6 units daily in pessaries. In nine patients it was given both topically (2×10^6 units daily) and by the intramuscular route (10^6 units daily). HLI was given for 21 days to all but one patient, who was treated for 40 days. The specific activity of HLI for topical application was 10^4 units and for intramuscular administration 5×10^4 units/mg. In two of the 15 patients grade IA malignancy was diagnosed, in ten patients grade IB, and in three patients grade IIB, according to the classification of the Fédération Internationale de Gynecologie et d'Obstetrique (FIGO). Histologically squamous-cell carcinoma was diagnosed in 14 patients and cervical polyp with malignant change in one.

Results after Therapy (Table II)

In three out of 15 patients with invasive cervical carcinoma (patients 10, 12, 14) tumor cells were not found in surgical material. In patient 15, who had invasive carcinoma (IB) before therapy, microinvasive carcinoma was identified after surgery; in two patients with invasive carcinoma (2 and 6) carcinoma-in-situ was identified in surgical material. In nine patients the findings were unchanged. Thus 40% of patients showed no carcinoma or a lower grade of carcinoma after HLI.

After application of HLI the papillary appearance of the tumor's surface disappeared and it became smooth and covered with fibrous membrane. In almost all patients the tumors developed a sharp distinction between tumor mass and healthy tissue, manifested in the formation of a fibrous wall. Bleeding from tumors diminished or stopped.

172   D. IKIĆ

TABLE II

Histological Findings on Biopsy of HLI-Treated Cervical-Cancer Patients

No.	Age	Histology Before HLI	Histology After HLI	Stromal reaction Before HLI	Stromal reaction After HLI	Assessment of general reactivity	Duration of the reactivity (days)	Adjuvant therapy
1	51	CIN	CIN	++	++	Poor	21	XRT
2	56	CIN	CIS	0	++++	Very good	21	-
3	33	CIN	CIN	+++	++++	Excellent	21	XRT
4	47	CIN	CIV	++++	+++	Moderate	21	XRT
5	43	CIN	CIN	+++	+	Poor	21	XRT
6	35	CIN	CIS	+++	++++	Excellent	21	-
7	39	CIN	CIN	+++	+++	Very good	40	XRT
8	35	CIN	CIV	+++	+++	Very good	21	XRT
9	38	CIN	CIN	+++	+++	Very good	21	XRT
10	48	CIM	NoCa	++	++++	Excellent	21	-
11	24	CIN	CIV	+++	+++	Very good	21	XRT
12	55	CIN	NoCa	+	+++	Excellent	21	-
13	55	CIN	CIN	+++	+	No response	21	XRT
14	23	CIM	NoCa	+++	+++	Excellent	21	-
15	29	CIN	CIM	+++	+++	Excellent	21	XRT

Histology: CIM = microinvasive carcinoma; CIN = invasive carcinom; CIS = carcinoma in situ; CIV = carcinoma in blood vessels; NoCa = no carcinoma; XRT = irradiation.

Stromal Reaction: No reaction = 0; Poor = +; Moderate = ++; Strong = +++; Very strong = ++++

Our investigations into the treatment of cervical carcinoma with HLI have been conducted in three phases, and 37 patients have been treated. There was not one case of tumor progression during HLI therapy, and in almost all patients the tumor mass was reduced by a third of its initial size. There was no difference in the results of therapy between patients who had received topical HLI only and those who had been given both topical and intramuscular HLI.

HEAD AND NECK TUMORS

As a result of laboratory and clinical investigations carried out in Zagreb in the past ten years (Ikić et al., 1975), perilesional and intralesional application of crude HLI was introduced in 1977 for treatment of a group of patients with head and neck tumors (Ikić et al., 1976). We have investigated the effect of interferon on skin tumors for the following reasons:

(a) Clinical observations of the process and verification of the diagnosis and treatment results are simple and objectively measurable.

(b) Injection of interferon into a skin tumor, and the surrounding area is simple and harmless.

(c) Removal of the tissue for biopsy is easy.

(d) Skin cancers are fairly common.

(e) Experience in Zagreb has shown that local infiltration of interferon into the tumor and the surrounding area stimulates immune reaction at the site of the lesion.

Patients and Methods

30 patients with cancer were treated with interferon. There were 12 women and 18 men, aged 44 to 91. The sites of the tumors were: cheek and chin 3, lower lip 5, nose 7, forehead 4, ear shell 3, neck 2, tonsil 3 and tongue 1. One patient had tumors in several sites, and one had a benign skin tumor.

The duration of HLI treatment was one to six months, depending on the clinical course of the disease. Interferon was administered by injection into the tumor or the surrounding area. During the first seven - 19 days interferon was administered daily and then two or three times weekly. A single daily dose was 3×10^5 units of non-purified interferon. In some of the cases an ointment containing 3×10^4 units HLI/g was applied.

The patient with tongue cancer, who had previously laryngeal carcinoma, was given therapy with 5×10^5 units twice daily intramuscularly as well as local infiltration in the area of the tongue.

Histologically, there were 13 cases of squamous-cell carcinoma, 15 of basal-cell carcinoma, one of neurogenic sarcoma, and one of benign skin tumor.

Since both diagnosis and objective evaluation of tumor and host cellular immunity are based on histological findings, exploratory biopsy was performed in all patients before the start of treatment.

Biopsies were examined histologically and in some cases histochemically. Results of treatment were evaluated by means of clinical observations during the course of HLI application and the microscopical appearance of the tumor or the tumor residue on completion of treatment.

Results

Local administration of HLI produced substantial or total remissions in patients with cancer of the head and neck. At the end of HLI therapy ten of 30 patients were considered completely cured. In ten patients unepithelialised skin lesions were hardly visible, in five the tumors were significantly reduced in size and had clear-cut borders, in two the tumors showed a tendency towards regression, and in three there was no effect. In some cases, severe mutilation of patients was avoided. Application of HLI close to the tumor site appears to prevent dispersal of tumor cells during surgical removal of the tumor. It also inhibited metastatic spread, thereby reducing the likelihood of recurrence.

URINARY BLADDER PAPILLOMATOSIS

Eight patients (five women and three men) with malignant recurrent papillomatosis of the urinary bladder had been treated repeatedly with transurethral resection and coagulation. Recurrences occurred three to eleven times at intervals of one to six months. Three patients in whom electroresection did not produce remission were given irradiation, but this also failed to control the disease. Biopsy material for histological and histochemical examination was removed before HLI therapy, three weeks after completion, and in the advanced stage of tumor regression. HLI was applied transurethrally with a surgical cystoscope once a day for 21 days. HLI (2×10^6 units) was injected into the tumor base or the surrounding tissue; and where the site of tumor would not permit this, HLI was injected into the wall of the urinary bladder as near the tumor as possible. In two patients interferon was simultaneously given by intramuscular injection at a dose of 2×10^6 units daily. The treatment was repeated at monthly intervals until the tumor regressed. In two patients the papillomas were reduced with electroresection after the first HLI administration.

One male and three female patients with bladder papillomatosis showed complete regression of tumors within three months of the beginning of therapy with HLI alone (Table III). In two women with diffuse papillomatosis and severe haematuria the beginning of regression, which was observed only after the third and fourth cycles of HLI therapy respectively, allowed transurethral electroresection, which had not previously been possible. This combined therapy led to a complete regression in both patients, 14 and 16 months respectively from the beginning of HLI therapy. In patient seven a striking regression has been observed during HLI therapy and is continuing. In patient three a complete regression was recorded after two months therapy. However, recurrence occurred after four months, and repeated HLI failed to produce any therapeutic effect.

Comparison of biopsy specimens removed before and during HLI application showed that the papillomas had lost their proliferative epithelium and were covered with atrophic inert epithelium. The stroma of the tumor showed severe proliferative inflammation and numerous lymphocytes and macrophages.

Recurrent papillomatosis which is not cured by electroresection and radiation progresses to disseminated disease and death. Because cystectomy is a severely mutilating procedure, HLI is now used in patients with urinary-bladder papillomatosis in whom conventional treatments had failed. Similar observations were described by Oberiter et al. (1979) in eight patients and Vuckovíc et al. (1979) in four patients.

BREAST CANCER

In four patients with breast cancer (two with primary carcinoma and two with recurrence) 2×10^6 i.u. interferon was injected into the lesion daily and 10^6 i.u. given intramuscularly daily for 60 days. When the tumor had regressed by more than 50% it was resected. The patients were given further HLI at a dose of 2×10^6 i.m. units three times weekly for six months.

Topical application of interferon led to more than 50% tumor regression in all four patients studied. The tumors did not metastasise during HLI therapy. In one patient an inflammatory carcinoma was subsequently resected having been inoperable prior to therapy. Local recurrence was not observed, but the patient died from distant metastases. In another patient, who refused mastectomy, the tumor diminished by 50% and was then excised. In all four patients HLI had an effect not only on the tumor itself, but also on the axillary lymph nodes, which enlarged during HLI therapy and returned to normal size after its withdrawal. The appearance of the lymph nodes during HLI application suggested lymphadenitis. Such changes could be misinterpreted as metastatic spread of the tumor to the lymph nodes.

TABLE III

Treatment of Bladder Papillomatosis with HLI and Standard Therapy

Patient No.	Sex	Age	No. of recur-rences	Papil-loma grade	Previous Treatment	Topical	i.m.	Duration of the therapy (mo)	Complete regres-sion	Adjuvant therapy	Duration if re-mission (mo)
1	F	75	3	II	3x electro-resection	42	-	3	Yes	-	32*
2	F	53	5	I	4x electro-resection	21	-	2	Yes	-	29
3	M	42	3	II	electro-resection	42	-	3	Yes	-	4
4	F	56	7	II	electro-resection	21	-	1	Yes	-	25
5	F	68	2	II	electro-resection	62	104	6	Yes	electro-resection	36
6	F	65	4	II	electro-resection and XRT	60	120	4	Yes	electro-resection	46
7	M	54	11	II	Resection, electro-resection and XRT	120	28	2	Yes	-	16†
8	M	52	2	II	electro-resection	120	28	2	Yes	-	22

* Died of heart attack; † Cystectomy.

TABLE IV

Breast Cancer – Intrapleural Treatment with HLI

No.	Age	Primary Treatment	Sites of Metastases	Application of HLI		Cytology after Treatment
				No.	Days	
1	25	XRT	pleura, soft tissues, lung, brain	2	1,2	–
2	70	S	pleura, soft tissues	5	1,4,8,11,13	No mal. cells after 3rd application
3	53	XRT	pleura, soft tissues	6	1,5,8,20,33, 76	No mal. cells after 4th application
4	55	S	pleura	4	1,5,10,12	No mal. cells (biopsy)
5	49	S	pleura	4	1,3,8,12	No mal. cells after 2nd application
6	38	XRT	pleura, liver, bone	2	1,6	degeneration after 2nd application

XRT = Radiotherapy; S = Surgery.

Pleural Effusions

Human leukocyte interferon was given into the pleural cavity in
six patients with breast cancer who had unilateral pleural effusions.
All patients were previously treated for their primary tumor either
by surgery or radiotherapy; whilst for their recurrent disease they
received either hormones, chemotherapy or both. All had developed a
second relapse when they were chosen for treatment with HLI. In all
patients' chest X-ray revealed pleural effusion and the diagnosis of
malignancy was confirmed by cytological or histological examination.
Response to treatment was evaluated by cytological examination of the
pleural fluid on each application. Malignant cells disappeared after
the second, third or fourth application, whilst the effusion
persisted (Jereb et al., 1977).

The number of malignant cells decreased successively while
histiocytes, and macrophages appeared and the number of leukocytes
increased. After the malignant cells completely disappeared and the
treatment was discontinued, the number of non-malignant cells began
to decrease. The total number and timing of interferon installation
are shown for each patient in Table VI.

CONDYLOMATA ACUMINATA

HLI was applied to treat condylomata acuminata or genital warts
in women. Pilot studies with HLI have shown that in 90% of patients
the complete regression of these benign tumors of skin and mucous
membranes takes eight weeks at the longest (Table V).

The therapeutic effect of HLI was evaluated in a double-blind
placebo-controlled clinical trial, which was carried out in ten pairs
of women with condylomata of various sizes, duration, and

TABLE V

Effect of Topical Use of HLI Ointment on
Condylomata Acuminata in 40 Women

Clinical findings after completed therapy with HPI	Patient No.	Duration of therapy with HLI (weeks)						
		2	3	4	5	6	7	8
Complete regression	36	1	2	12	6	8	6	1
Unchanged	4				3			1

TABLE VI

Effect of HLI and Placebo on Condylomata Acuminata
Within Pairs of Treated Women*

Pair	Interferon	Placebo	Difference within a pair in 5th week of therapy**
	Regression (weeks)	Regression (weeks)	
1	4	3	0
2	5	4	0
3	10	none	1
4	12	none	1
5	4	none	1
6	5	6	0
7	12	none	1
8	12	none	1
9	9	none	1
10	9	none	1

*
    Comparison of the therapeutic effect within pairs
    $p = 0.007$ (Wilcoxon two-sample sign test for the paired case).

**
    0 = No difference in effect between HLI and placebo;
    1 = Marked effect of HLI in comparison with placebo.

localization. Each woman of the pair received either HLI or placebo
in the form of ointment that was to be topically applied four to five
times daily in the course of five weeks (Table VI). This period of
time was chosen on the basis of the experience gained in pilot trials
in which we demonstrated therapeutic benefit of HLI on C.A. In four
patients treated with HLI (4,000 units/g), complete regression took
place, whereas in the other six patients the condylomata decreased in
size and therefore the HLI therapy was continued until complete
regression occured after nine, ten and 12 weeks from the beginning of
therapy. In ten women receiving placebo, complete regression took
place in two cases after three and four weeks, respectively, whereas
in one case the size of the condylomata decreased after five weeks so
that placebo was further administered until its disappearance one
week later. In the remaining seven women of the group treated, no
regression occurred. The therapeutic effect of HLI was statistically
significant when compared to placebo. Of the seven women given
placebo with no success, only five came for further treatment with

HLI. In all five women, complete regression of genital warts took place after four, eight and 12 weeks of HLI treatment (Ikić et al., 1981; Ikić et al., 1975).

CONCLUSIONS

We have used human leukocyte interferon which has been concentrated, but not purified. The application has been intra-lesional, perilesional or topical, and the dose of interferon modest.

None of the patients studied had noeplasms that improve spontaneously and the results provide evidence that the disease was favorably influenced by the treatment given. Of course, many questions remain unanswered. Would the apparent "cures" persist? Would the same effect be produced by more refined material? How was the effect produced - by a direct effect on tumor cells, or through the stromal response?

We believe that the administration of HLI results in an increased lymphocyte and macrophage infiltrate within tumors. These cells showed signs of enhanced destructive activity towards the tumor. The response in the regional lymph nodes has also been stimulated.

It is important to point out that the administration of HLI does not induce any specific response which would not otherwise be present in the normal interaction of stroma and parenchyma of a carcinoma. HLI accelerates, enhances and protracts the interaction between stroma and carcinoma. We are continuing to evaluate the histological and clinical responses of accessible tumors to HLI.

REFERENCES

Ikić, D., Krusić, J., Cupak, K., Car, D., Rogulguić, A., Jakasa, V., Jusić, D., Soos, E. and Turner, V. 1975, The use of human leukocytic interferon in patients with cervical cancer and baseocellular cancer of the skin, in: "Proc. Symp. Clinical Use of Interferon", 9th Int. Immunobiol. Symp., D. Ikić, ed., Yugoslav Academy of Sciences and Arts, Zagreb, 239.
Ikić, D., Beck, M., Turner, V., Soos, E., Lulić, V. and Jusić, D. 1976, An in vitro testing of LED-Widr cell invasiveness inhibition in the presence of interferon, in: "Proc. Symp. Stability and Effectiveness Measles, Poliomyelitis, Pertussis Vaccines", 10th Int. Immunobiol. Symp., D. Ikić, ed., Yugoslav Academy of Sciences and Arts, Zagreb, 247.
Ikić, D., Nola, P., Maricić, Z., Smud, K., Oresić, V., Knezević, M., Rode, B., Jusić, D. and Soos, E. 1981a, Application of human leukocyte interferon in patients with urinary bladder papillomatotis, breast cancer, and melanoma, Lancet, 1:1022.

Ikić, D., Krusić, J., Kirmajer, V., Knezević, M., Maricić, Z., Rode, B., Jusić, D. and Soos, E. 1981b, Application of human leukocyte interferon in patients with carcinoma of the uterine cervix, Lancet, 1:1027.

Ikić, D., Trajer, D., Cupak, K., Petricevic, I., Prasić, M., Soldo, I., Jusić, D., Smerdel, S. and Soos, E. 1981c, The clinical use of human leukocyte interferon in viral infections, Inter. J. Clin. Pharmacology, Therapy and Toxicology, 10:498.

Ikić, D., Singer, Z., Beck, M., Soos, E., Sips, D. and Jusić, D. 1981d, Interferon treatment of uterine cervical precancerosis, J. Cancer Res. Clin. Oncol., 101:303.

Jereb, B., Cervek, J., Krasovec, U., Ikić, D. and Soos, E. 1977, Intrapleural application of human leukocyte interferon (HLI) in breast cancer patients with unilateral pleural carcinosis. Preliminary report, in: "Proc. Symp. Preparation, Standardization and Clinical Use of Interferon", 11th Int. Immunobiol. Symp., D. Ikić, Yugoslav Academy of Sciences and Arts, Zagreb, 187.

Krusić, J., Ikić, D., Knezević, M., Soos, E., Rode, B., Jusić, D. and Maricić, Z. 1977, Clinical and histological findings after local application of human leukocyte interferon in patients with cervical cancer, in: "Proc. Symp. Preparation, Standardization and Clinical Use of Interferon", 11th Int. Immunobiol. Symp., D. Ikić, ed., Yugoslav Academy of Sciences and Arts, Zagreb, 167.

Oberiter, B., Kraljić, I., Knezević, M. and Ikić, D. 1979, Prva iskustva u terapiji interferonom kod papiloma i papilarnih tumora mokraćnog mjehura, in: "Zbornik radova Savjetovanja o bolnickim ispitivanjima interferona", Interferon i tumori, D. Ikić, ed., JAZU, Zagreb, 110.

Vucković, I., Matulić, S. and Soos, E. 1979, Utjecaj humanog leukocitnog interferona na recidivne tumore mokraćnog mjehura, in: "Zbornik radova Savjetovanja o klinickim ispitivanjima interferona", Interferon i tumori, D. Ikić, ed., JAZU, Zagreb, 114.

CLINICAL TRIALS OF INTERFERON INDUCERS

ARTHUR S. LEVINE AND STEPHEN A. SHERWIN

Division of Cancer Treatment, National Cancer Institute
Bethesda, Maryland 20205, U.S.A.

INTERFERON INDUCTION IN MAN

Initial attempts to exploit the potential antitumor activity of
interferon in man were dependent on the induction of endogenous
interferon by a variety of agents. In recent years, the increasing
availability and study of exogenous interferon produced by
recombinant DNA methodology (as well as by large scale culture
techniques) has largely replaced this effort. Moreover, there are
certain limitations in the clinical usefulness of interferon inducers
including a relatively high degree of toxicity and low therapeutic
index, hyporeactivity to repeated induction, and potential antibody
formation against the inducer itself. Despite these limitations, a
review of the cancer clinical trials conducted to date with
interferon inducers should prove instructive in the future development and interpretation of exogenous interferon studies in man.

The subject of interferon inducers has been previously reviewed
(Beers and Braun, 1971; Finter, 1973; Ho and Armstrong, 1975, Levy
and Levine, 1982; Stringfellow, 1980). Type 1 interferons (alpha and
beta) are best induced by double-stranded RNA, found in viruses in
their native or replicative forms, or produced chemically as
synthetic polynucleotides. Less effective inducers of these
interferons include various intracellular micro-organisms and
microbial cell wall products; synthetic polymers including pyran
copolymers; and a variety of miscellaneous low molecular weight
substances including tilorone, propanediamine, acranil, dibenzyl-
furan, kanamycin, and cycloheximide. This list of interferon
inducers has been largely generated from in vitro and animal studies.
Preliminary clinical trials in man have for the most part focused on
synthetic polynucleotides including poly IC, poly ICLC, and poly

183

A-poly U. Only very limited and inconclusive in vivo testing has
been carried out to date with interferon inducers belonging to the
other categories listed above. Many of the interferon inducers
identified in in vitro studies have proved to be too toxic to test
extensively in man.

Poly A-poly U is a synthetic double-stranded complex of poly-
adenylic and polyuridylic acid. Poly A-poly U is a relatively poor
inducer of interferon and may exert its clinical effects on the basis
of other mechanisms involving the immune system. For example, poly
A-poly U can stimulate antibody synthesis in both normal and immuno-
deficient mice (Schmidtke and Johnson, 1971), and can also stimulate
the cellular immune system as evidenced by an improved capacity of
neonatally thymectomized mice to respond to skin allografts and an
increased degree of differentiation of T lymphocytes from precursor
cells in genetically athymic mice (Cone and Johnson, 1971; Scheid et
al., 1973). However, in early trials of poly A-poly U at the
Memorial Sloan-Kettering Cancer Center, in which patients with
disseminated cancer were immunologically monitored during treatment,
no clear pattern of immunologic enhancement was observed (Wanebo et
al., 1976). Changes in skin test reactivity were variable. In vitro
responsiveness of T lymphocytes was decreased to mitogens and
increased to specific antigens (especially if pretreatment reactivity
had been depressed), whereas peripheral T lymphocyte counts were
decreased after poly A-poly U treatment. Although the immunologic
mechanisms of action of poly A-poly U remain to be fully defined,
initial in vivo experiments did suggest anti- tumor activity in
various experimental animal models. Thus, poly A-poly U therapy was
shown to delay the appearance of spontaneous leukemia in AKR mice
(Drake et al., 1974), as well as to decrease the incidence of
spontaneous mammary tumors in C3H/He mice and transplantable melanoma
in hamsters (Lacour et al., 1972; Lacour et al., 1975).

Clinical trials of poly A-poly U in cancer patients have been
limited. Lacour and colleagues have recently reported the results of
a randomized trial in which poly A-poly U was administered as
adjuvant therapy to patients with operable breast cancer following
mastectomy (Lacour et al., 1982a; Lacour et al., 1982b). This trial
was conducted between 1972 and 1979 at the Institute Gustave-Roussy.
Three hundred patients were entered on the trial; 155 patients were
randomized to receive 30 mg of poly A-poly U intravenously once
weekly for six weeks, and 145 patients served as controls. All
patients had T-2 primary tumors with or without lymph node involvement. Patients with positive lymph nodes were given postoperative
radiation therapy as well as a radiotherapeutic oophorectomy.
Toxicity was limited to minimal temperature elevation in only 20 of
the 155 treated patients. A statistically significant improvement in
five-year actuarial survival was reported for the poly A-poly U
treated group. An even greater improvement in five-year relapse-free
actuarial survival was reported in the poly A-poly U treated patients

with positive lymph nodes (71% vs. 47% in he untreated controls). These encouraging results require confirmation; moreover, the mechanism of action of poly A-poly U in these patients is not clear and there was no demonstrable increase in serum interferon activity in the treated patients. There are no trials reported to date in which poly A-poly U has been tested on patients with advanced metastatic tumors.

Clinical trials of interferon inducers other than synthetic poly-nucleotides have been very fragmentary (Merigan and Regelson, 1967; Morahan et al., 1978; Pavilides et al., 1978; Stolfi and Martin, 1978). Tilorone is a water soluble dicyclic amine which can be orally administered. Although tilorone can induce interferon in laboratory animals, it does not appear to do so in man in doses that are well-tolerated, and no definite in vivo immuno-modulatory effects have been identified (Niblack, 1977). Tilorone has been shown to be active against virally-induced and transplantable rodent tumors including Friend leukemia, L1210, and Lewis Lung Carcinoma (Regelson, 1976). However, despite an early report of transient antitumor activity in two patients with melanoma (Wampler et al., 1973), phase II efficacy trials of tilorone at the Medical College of Virginia involving 66 patients with melanoma and a variety of other cancers failed to demonstrate any consistent antitumor activity (Regelson, 1976). Moreover, these early trials of tilorone have revealed definite dose-limiting gastrointestinal and CNS toxicity, as well as significant ocular toxicity (Regelson, 1976; Wampler et al., 1973).

MVE-2 is a pyran copolymer consisting of divinyl ether and maleic anhydride which has been shown to have in vivo antitumor activity against spontaneous and transplanted tumors in mice (Morahan et al., 1978; Stolfi and Martin, 1978). Although previously shown to induce interferon in mice, MVE-2 is now thought to exert its anti-tumor activity on the basis of macrophage activation (Pavilides et al., 1978). An early clinical trial of this agent in patients with disseminated cancer demonstrated increased endogenous interferon activity, but no antitumor effect was reported (Merigan and Regelson, 1967). The National Cancer Institute has recently sponsored phase I clinical trials of this agent, the results of which will be reported in the near future.

POLY IC AND POLY ICLC: TOXICITY TRIALS

The inducers most extensively studied in clinical trials are poly IC and poly ICLC, and the remainder of this chapter will be devoted to a review of these studies. The synthetic double-stranded RNA, poly I-poly C, is an effective inducer of interferon in vitro and in vivo (Beers and Braun, 1971; Buckler et al., 1971; Field et al., 1967; Field et al., 1972; Finter, 1973; Hilleman, 1968), and has proven to be useful in prophylaxis and treatment of lytic viral infections in rodents (Catalano and Baron, 1970; Field et al., 1967; Kern et al., 1975). As with interferon (Glasgow et al., 1978; Gresser, 1977; Gresser et al., 1978; Gresser and Tovey, 1978), there is evidence that poly I-poly C may have, in addition to an antiviral role, an antineoplastic action. The compound has been success- fully to inhibit the growth of various transplantable rodent tumors, including those known to be induced by virus and those that are apparently spontaneous in origin (Sarma et al., 1969; Zeleznick and Bhuyan, 1969; Levy et al., 1970; Kreider and Benjamin, 1972; Levy, 1977). The polynucleotide has at least three activities that might be related to its antitumor activity: (a) induction of interferon; (b) non-specific stimulation of immune mechanisms; and (c) non-specific and specific effects on cell membranes and on macro- molecular synthesis (Beers and Braun, 1971; Kreider and Benjamin, 1972; Finter, 1973; Gresser, 1977; Gresser et al., 1978; Gresser and Tovey, 1978). While poly I-poly C is a good interferon inducer as well as an effective antiviral and antitumor agent in rodents, it is a poor interferon inducer in humans and is not clinically useful at any dosage (Robinson et al., 1976). Rapid hydrolysis in human serum appears to be responsible for the absence of activity (Nordlund et al., 1970).

A stabilized poly I-poly C complex, poly ICLC, has been prepared by Levy et al. which appears to resist hydrolysis by serum nuclease and is an effective interferon inducer in subhuman primates (Levy et al., 1975; Purcell et al., 1976). The stabilized product is a complex of high molecular weight poly I-poly C and low molecular weight poly-L-lysine. The preparation, which also contains carboxy- methylcellulose, protects rhesus monkeys against otherwise lethal viral infections (Levy, 1977; Levy et al., 1975; Levy et al., 1976; Purcell et al., 1976). Extensive toxicologic studies have been completed in rodents, cats, rhesus monkeys, and chimpanzees (Levine et al., 1979).

Recently, initial clinical trials of poly ICLC in cancer patients were reported; these reports established an approximate maximum tolerable dose in humans, and characterized dose-response curves for interferon induction in the serum and cerebrospinal fluid (Levine et al., 1979; Levine et al., 1981; Levine et al., 1982; Levy and Levine, 1982). The emphasis of these trials has been on patients with actue leukemia, lymphoma, multiple myeloma, and juvenile laryngeal papillomatosis. These tumors were chosen for studies of clinical efficacy because they are among those diseases described in preliminary reports as demonstrating a response to purified (exogenous) human interferon per se (Einhorn and Strander, 1977; Hill et al., 1979; Mellstedt et al., 1979; Merigan et al., 1978; Skurkivich et al., 1977).

In an initial (phase I) toxicity trial, poly ICLC was administered to 25 patients, all of whom had solid tumors or acute

TABLE I

Mean Peak Serum Interferon Titers
After Treatment with Poly ICLC

Dose Level (mg/m^2)	Mean Reference units/ml[a]
0.5	15 (0-25)[b]
2.5	15 (0-25)
7.5	198 (25-250)
12.0	1,940 (200-5,000)
18.0	4,473 (600-15,000)
27.0	5,820 (2,000-10,143)

[a]VSV/CPE assay (international reference units); sample taken 8 hr after first dose; $\geq$ 3 trials at each level.

[b]Range is given in parentheses.

similar. The mean peak serum interferon titers attained in this trial were extraordinarily high, exceeding those usually noted with naturally occuring viral infections. The correlation between drug dose and peak interferon titer was approximately linear.

In the initial phase I trial, the maximum tolerated dose for all patients at a given drug dose was found to be about 12 mg/m^2. In general, the 25 patients included in this study were quite stable and had relatively limited disease (Levine et al., 1979). Subsequent experience has shown that in patients who have more extensive disease, have constitutional symptoms, or are at the extremes of age, the maximum tolerated dose of poly ICLC appears to be less than 12 mg/m^2 (Krown et al., 1981; and as will be described below). At the 12 mg/m^2 dose, the mean peak serum interferon titer was 1940 reference units/ml. Poly ICLC also induced interferon in the cerebrospinal fluid when given intravenously; however, the peak interferon titers obtained were considerably less than those noted in the serum (Table II). Of the CSF samples collected, the eight hr sample following the first dose of poly ICLC demonstrated the highest titer in all patients. It should be noted that a very broad range of serum interferon titers was found at every dose level, suggesting considerable individual variation in response to this drug or its metabolism.

The most frequently encountered toxic reaction in the initial phase I trial of poly ICLC (Levine et al., 1979) was fever, which occurred in 100% of clinical trials and did not abate significantly leukemia refractory to established therapy (Levine et al., 1979). At least three complete clinical trials were conducted at each of six dose levels within the range 0.5 - 27.0 mg/m^2. Each patient was treated at only one dose level. The drug was given intravenously over a 60 min period on the first day of the study, followed by a seven-day rest period to permit evaluation of any unanticipated toxicity. Following the rest period, the drug was given every day for the next two weeks. The final preparation of poly ICLC contained 2 mg poly I-poly C/ml and 1.5 mg poly-L-lysine/ml in 0.5% carboxy-methylcellulose.

Toxicity evaluation was based on hemogram, liver studies, renal function, coagulation studies, serum chemistry determinations, and a bromsulfophthalein test of liver function. All of these studies were performed before the first dose of poly ICLC and were repeated 24 and 48 hr after the initial dose. Thereafter, studies were done once, twice or three times weekly (as appropriate) for the duration of each patient's study. Appropriate serial studies (X-ray examination, radioisotope scans, bone marrow aspirates and biopsies, and tumor markers) were carried out to assess tumor response, with weekly estimates of tumor mass.

Serum interferon concentrations were determined on samples collected immediately prior to the drug infusion on day one; subsequent samples were collected eight and 24 hr after the start of the one hr infusion. To determine interferon titers, the VSV/CPE protection test was used (Oie et al., 1972). One unit of interferon is defined as that amount which, when suitably incubated with proper test cells, will cause a reduction of 0.5 $\log_{10}$ in the yield of a suitable sensitive challenge virus (VSV) as compared with the yield from cells not treated with interferon (CPE). Interferon titers are expressed as reference units per milliliter.

Table I lists the mean peak serum interferon titers attained following administration of poly ICLC at a dose range of 0.5 - 27.0 mg/m^2. In preliminary trials, with serum sampled every four hr for 24 hr following each dose, peak levels were noted in the sample collected eight hr after the first dose of poly ICLC; the tabulated data therefore represent the mean serum interferon titers at that time for all patients.

All patients had pretreatment levels of less than five reference units/ml. As noted with the parent compound, poly I-poly C, peak interferon levels dropped rapidly with continued daily exposure to the drug (Buckler et al., 1971; DuBuy et al., 1970; Robinson et al., 1976); at 7.5 mg/m^2, the mean peak interferon titer after the fifth dose was 50 reference units/ml. Representative kinetic curves of interferon induction in response to the parent compound, poly I-poly C, have been published (Robinson et al., 1976), and the kinetics of serum interferon in response to each and all doses of poly ICLC were

TABLE II

Mean Peak Cerebrospinal Fluid Interferon Titers
After Treatment with Poly ICLC

Dose Level (mg/m^2)	Means Reference units/ml[a]
0.5	5 (0–10)[b]
12.0	34 (5–63)
18.0	55 (0–115)
27.0	515 (79–1000)

[a] VSV/CPE assay; sample taken eight hr after first dose; $\geq$ 3 trials at each level.

[b] Range is given in parentheses.

with continued exposure to the drug (Table III). The mean peak temperature elevation was 1.5°C, which usually occurred four – eight hr after drug administration and persisted for approximately six – 12 hr. No relation was found between the development of fever and the dose level or magnitude of interferon induction. Nausea, modest elevations of liver enzyme levels, thrombocytopenia, and leukopenia were noted less consistently. No relationship was found between the dose level or magnitude of induction and the toxic hematologic manifestations. Moreover, in many cases the findings could not be ascribed to exposure to the drug per se, as opposed to the consequences of the underlying disease. It does seem likely that the drug produces peripheral cytopenia due to destruction or sequestration. Moreover, a subtle arrest of marrow maturation cannot be excluded.

The most significant toxicities noted in the phase I trial were those of hypotension and a syndrome of polyarthralgia and polymyalgia. These side effects did relate to dose level and/or the magnitude of interferon induction, unlike the other toxic manifestations. Interestingly, in those patients who experienced a moderate decrease in blood pressure, the pressure tended to stabilize or increase during continued exposure to the drug. The syndrome of polyarthralgia and polymyalgia was often accompanied by erythema over the tender joints, and usually occurred after three to five doses in the 12–18 mg/m2 dose range. The picture was consistent with a serum sickness–like reaction, and in three of the four patients who experienced this syndrome, symptoms and signs began to decrease while the drug was continued. In the four patients who developed the serum sickness–like syndrome, an attempt was made to detect serum antibody to poly I–poly C using a Farr–type technique (Steinberg et al.,

TABLE III

Poly ICLC Toxicity

Manifestation	No./total
Fever	25/25 (100)[a]
Nausea	11/25 (44)
Thrombocytopenia and leukopenia	17/25 (68)
Hypotension[b]	7/25 (28)
Syndrome of erythema, polyarthralgia, and polymyalgia[b]	4/25 (16)
Renal failure[b]	1/25 (4)
Trial aborted[c]	5/25 (20)

[a] Percentage is given in parentheses.

[b] Related to dose level and/or magnitude of interferon induction.

[c] Due to hypotension in three, renal failure (27 mg/m^2) in one, and ser sickness (?) in one. Maximum tolerated dose, 12 mg/m^2.

1969), but Farr-type polynucleotide antibodies could not be demonstrated in these patients.

In summary, the maximum tolerated dose for all patients at a given drug dose in the initial phase I trial was about 12 mg/m^2. At this dose, the mean peack serum interferon titer was 1940 reference units/ml. Five of 25 (20%) clinical trials had to be aborted because of toxicity, three due to clinically significant hypotension, one due to acute renal failure, and one due to severe polyarthralgia-polymyalgia (all five aborted trials were at a dose of 18 mg/m^2 or higher).

In the initial phase I trial, 23 of 25 patients demonstrated progressive tumor over a six-week period of observation (three weeks on study plus a subsequent three weeks of observation). However, one adult with acute undifferentiated leukemia demonstrated a brief period of stabilization, and one child with acute lymphoblastic leukemia appeared to enter a complete remission after treatment with poly ICLC. An interpretation of this child's response to the drug is complicated, however, by his exposure to a low dose of cyclophosphamide just prior to the poly ICLC trial (Levine et al., 1979).

POLY ICLC: TUMOUR ACTIVITY TRIALS

Following completion of the phase I toxicity study, summarized above, broad phase II studies of this highly effective interferon inducer were initiated.   The general plan of these studies is to employ the inducer in patients whose tumors are refractory to established therapy, with the exception of adults with acute myelocytic leukemia who are treated at the time of first relapse. Poly ICLC is given, except where noted, at the 12 mg/m^2 dose level every other day for 30 days.   If the patient demonstrates a complete, partial, or stable tumor response, he is maintained on the drug three times a week for up to 18 months.   Fifteen to 25 patients with each disease are to be studied, depending upon response rates.   A number of ancillary studies, including the effects of poly ICLC on natural killer cell activity and antibody-dependent cellular cytotoxicity, are also being conducted.

Trials sponsored by the National Cancer Institute emphasize acute leukemia, lymphoma, and sarcomas, and clinical results to date are shown in Table IV.   All of these patients received a 12 mg/m dose every other day.   There were no clinically useful tumor responses among these 25 patients, and it is again notable that peak interferon induction was widely variable.   There are not yet sufficient numbers of patients in any one disease category to draw a statistically significant conclusion regarding clinical efficacy of poly ICLC in any of these diseases.   Moreover, with the exception of the patients with acute myelocytic leukemia, all patients in these trials are resistant to established therapy and have been heavily pretreated with chemotherapy and/or radiotherapy.   Interestingly, the majority of these patients have shown a markedly enhanced natural killer cell activity during treatment (R.Herberman, et al., in preparation).

A larger number of patients with childhood acute leukemia have been enrolled in a trial of the Children's Cancer Study Group

TABLE IV

Results of NCI Phase II Trial of Poly ICLC

Disease	No. of patients	No. of doses	Peak interferon titer (units/ml)	Response
Acute lymphocytic leukemia	6	7–14	50–800	0
Acute myelocytic leukemia	6	6–30	30–794	1 PR[a], 1 stable
Burkitt's lymphoma	4	6–14	5–500	0
Osteosarcoma	6	7–26	200–1000	0
Hodgkin's disease	3	4–15	50–794	0

[a]PR: partial remission.

(Lampkin et al., 1982). All patients were in relapse after receiving all standard drugs. In initial studies in this patient population at 12 mg/m2, it was noted that toxicity was more severe than anticipated on the basis of the earlier phase I trial (with hypotension and arthralgia frequent, and CNS findings present infrequently). All of these children were ill at the time of the poly ICLC study, and the majority were very young (median age, eight), febrile, and had extensive disease. The increment in fever and stress produced by poly ICLC apparently rendered the drug less tolerable in virtually all children than had been the case in our initial trial, and the dosage for the CCSG trial has been reduced so that the starting level is now 3 mg/m2. At this starting dose, most children eventually tolerated 6-9 mg/m2.

At present, 37 children have been entered in this study, 20 of whom had null-type acute lymphoblastic leukemia (5,T-ALL; 3,AUL; 9;ANLL). Eighteen of the patients are evaluable for clinical response (an adequate trial consisted of 14 daily doses at the tolerated dose). The range of peak interferon titers for all dose levels was 10-1300 ref. units/ml. No complete remission was observed in the CCSG trial. However, five responses were noted, as shown in Table V. Thus, poly (ICLC) does have antileukemic activity, but the drug may be too toxic for end-stage patients.

In a study at the University of Arizona (Lampkin et al., 1982), patients with multiple myeloma and definitive evidence of disease

TABLE V

CCSG Trial in Childhood Leukemia: Response to Poly (ICLC)

Type of Leukemia	Dosage	#Days Given	BEFORE		AFTER	
			WBC	% Blasts	WBC	% Blasts
T Cell[*]	9 mg/m^2	14	91,600	95	100	0%
Null ALL	9 mg/m^2	14	18,850	99	25	60%
Null ALL	6 mg/m^2	14	140,000	94	900	0%
Null ALL	9 mg/m^2	14	77,000	96	100	24%
Null ALL[*]	9 mg/m^2	14	1,800	12	500	N.D.[**]

[*]   Bone marrow aspirate - no leukemia cells seen;
     Bone marrow biopsy - very hypocellular.

[**] Differential not done.

progression are receiving poly ICLC. All of these patients are no
longer responsive to conventional chemotherapy, and for entry into
the trial, it is required that they have demonstrated at least a 30%
increase in the serum M-component, a 50% increase in the urine
M-component (Bence Jones protein), and/or an increase in the size
and/or number of plasmacytomas or lytic bone lesions. Again, 15-25
patients with myeloma will be studied, depending upon the tumor
response rate. Poly ICLC is being administered for at least four
weeks, and until the disease progresses if there is a response or
stabilization. As with the study of childhood leukemia, the majority
of these patients have had advanced disease and were very ill (in
some cases, virtually moribund) at the time the trial was begun.
Here too, we have found the 12 mg/m^2 dose often intolerable (usually
because of severe rigors in patients who already have bone pain), and
the majority of the patients have been treated with 2-3 mg/m^2 after
the initial 12 mg dose. Moreover, in an attempt to circumvent the
hyporefractory state associated with all interferon inducers,
treatment is being given two to three times weekly as opposed to
daily; this schedule has also permitted treatment in the outpatient
clinic.

The results of the myeloma study to date are shown in Table VI.
Of the five patients shown, one (R.C.) has had a partial response and
two (J.K., J.S.) appear to have experienced some biologic effect
after treatment with poly ICLC. Effect is here defined mainly in
terms of the M-component, and there is not yet sufficient information
to determine the ultimate clinical meaning of these changes in the
M-component. It is noteworthy that at the 2-3 mg/m^2 dose, these
patients are maintaining serum interferon peaks of approximately
50-60 reference units/ml.

Other tumor activity trials of poly ICLC have been recently
initiated in patients with brain tumors, hepatoma, neuroblastoma,
colon carcinoma, melanoma, breast cancer, and Kaposi's sarcoma. The
results of these trials are not yet evaluable.

Finally, in a trial at the Johns Hopkins Hospital (Leventhal et
al., 1981), two children with juvenile laryngeal papillomatosis have
been studied. This rare disease, believed to be virus-induced and
often life-threatening due to airway obstruction, has previously been
reported to respond to purified exogenous human interferon (Einhorn
and Strander, 1977). The patients at Hopkins had both experienced
spread of the papillomatous process to involve the lower tracheobronchial tree and the lungs. Both received the 12 mg/m^2 dose three
times a week for at least five weeks, and tolerated this regimen
well, suggesting that patients with localized disease and no constitutional symptoms are able to tolerate this drug far more readily
than patients with advanced leukemia and similar disease processes.
One of these patients had required endoscopic surgery every four
weeks in order to maintain a patent airway. After the start of

TABLE VI

Results of Myeloma Study (University of Arizona Trial)

Patient	M-component	Treatment duration	Change in peak interferon titer[b] (units/ml)	change in M-component[b]	Clinical response	Toxicity
R.C.	Bence Jones	3+ mo	250 --> 60	20 --> 3g/ml	Symptoms decreased, no new bone lesions	Creatinine increased initially, later within normal limits
J.K.	IgG	7 wk	100 --> 50	5.5 -->3.5g/ml	Symptoms continued, lesions stable; IgG increased after trial	High fevers even with very low dose; neutropenia
J.S.	IgG	1 day	--> 600	2.9 -->1.2g/ml	After poly ICLC, responded to CV-BAP (had been refractory)	Hypertensive crisis
H.C.	IgG	3+ wk	300 --> 60	6.0 -->4.8g/ml	Too early	-
R.B.	Waldenstrom	2+ wk	250 --> 50	5.0 -->1.5g/ml	Too early	-

[a]Poly ICLC, 10-12 mg/m^2 initially, then 2-3 mg/m^2 two or three times weekly.
[b]Change from initial values to values at end of treatment.

treatment with poly ICLC, this child was maintained for 12 weeks
without surgery and with stable pulmonary disease. Treatment was
then discontinued, and surgery was required four weeks later, at
which time an increase in pulmonary disease was noted. The
interferon peak attained in this child was 1584 reference units/ml.
The second patient had required endoscopic surgery every two – three
weeks. After the start of poly ICLC, she was maintained for six
weeks without surgery. Further treatment was declined and the
disease recovered its previous momentum. The interferon peak in this
child was 2500 reference units/ml.

Discussion of Poly ICLC Trials

Poly ICLC, a polynucleotide interferon inducer stabilized so as
to make the complex resistant to hydrolysis by primate serum ribonuclease, was initially administered at dose levels of 0.5 – 27.0
mg/m^2 (with each patient treated at only one dose level). In adult
patients with limited disease and no constitutional symptoms, the
maximum tolerated dose was 12 mg/m^2. However, in patients at the
extremes of age, with extensive underlying disease, and/or with
constitutional symptoms, the additional stress associated with this
interferon inducer has usually rendered the 12 mg dose intolerable.
Preliminary results suggest that in the latter patient population, a
dose of approximately 2-3 mg/m^2 is tolerable except for fever,
although individual variation with respect to toxicity and interferon
induction continues to be broad at all dose levels. At all doses,
fever is the most common side effect. No patient has developed
significant abnormalities of liver function nor has any patient
experienced a marked disturbance of the clotting mechanism.
Peripheral cytopenia has been common, but only rarely has it been
possible to ascribe it to the drug exclusively, as opposed to the
underlying disease.

The clinically important toxicities that have so far been
observed include hypotension, acute renal failure, CNS findings, and
a syndrome of polyarthralgia-polymyalgia, primarily involving the
small joints. Unlike the other side effects, hypotension and
polyarthralgia-polymyalgia appear to be related to the dose level
and/or magnitude of interferon induction. It is not possible to
state whether these toxic manifestations are due to the poly ICLC
complex per se, to the high levels of endogenous interferon induced
by this drug, or both.

The fact that interferon is also induced in the cerebrospinal
fluid suggests the possible utility of poly ICLC in the management of
viral infections of the central nervous system such as rabies. The
possible use of poly ICLC in non-life-threatening viral infections
(central nervous system or systemic) must, of course, be balanced
against possible toxicity and the hyporesponsive phenomenon which
results in diminishing interferon levels with repeated exposure to
inducers.

The initial study of poly ICLC (Levine, et al., 1979) was designed to obtain phase I toxicity data and to generate a dose-response curve for interferon induction in humans. Only one or two patients with any given tumor type were exposed to the higher drug doses. While conclusions could not be drawn with respect to the antitumor efficacy of poly ICLC, the finding of one child with acute lymphocytic leukemia entering complete remission following exposure to poly ICLC was of particular interest in view of recent reports of bone marrow clearing of leukemic blasts following administration of human leukocyte interferon (Hill et al., 1979). Despite the fact that this response could not be assigned unambiguously, the CCSG undertook trials of poly ICLC in a larger number of patients with childhood acute lymphocytic leukemia. While antileukemic responses have been seen in the CCSG trials, it seems unlikely at the present time that poly ICLC will prove to have a significant (durable) antileukemic effect. This conclusion, of course, does not exclude the possibility that the inducer (or purified interferon) might be effective at an earlier point in the natural history of acute leukemia and when the tumor burden is low.

The results in multiple myeloma are of particular interest (Table VI) - although only a few patients have so far been studied - since patients with this disease have been reported in preliminary trials to show a response to purified human interferon. The decrements in M-component that have been observed in response to poly ICLC are of the same order of magnitude as seen with exogenous interferon (Mellstedt et al., 1979), but in both cases it is difficult at this time to render a definitive interpretation of the results. It is possible that the M-component has been decreased because of an increased catabolic rate or changes in plasma volume rather than because of an absolute decrease in the synthesis of the protein. It is also possible that even if the synthetic rate of the M-component is being reduced by treatment with interferon or interferon inducers, the proliferation of the myeloma cells per se has not been affected. Finally, since this is a steroid-responsive disease, a trivial explanation for the results might be steroid induction as a consequence of treatment with interferon or with the inducer. Nonetheless, these myeloma results are clearly of biologic interest. Whether they are of therapeutic interest as well will only be determined in more extensive studies. Intuitively, these studies should emphasize the use of interferon or the inducer as adjuvant therapy following the first chemotherapy-induced remission.

Finally, although only a small number of children with juvenile laryngeal papillomatosis have so far been treated, it is of considerable interest that the results have been similar to those reported with purified human interferon in the treatment of this rare disease (Einhorn and Strander, 1977), in that these patients have been able to tolerate longer surgery-free intervals while maintaining a patent airway.

Summary

A diversity of synthetic polymers, microbial products, and miscellaneous low-molecular weight substances have been studied as potential interferon inducers in cancer patients. Most such agents did not induce interferon at tolerable doses, and where very preliminary and unconfirmed results suggested some clinical anti-tumor efficacy, it was not at all clear that this was due to interferon induction. However, it has been established that poly ICLC, a nuclease-resistant synthetic polynucleotide, is the first highly effective and tolerable interferon inducer in humans. The tolerable dose range is between 2 and 12 mg/m^2 (with broad individual variations), depending upon age, extent of underlying disease, and presence of constitutional symptoms prior to treatment. When poly ICLC has been given more than once or twice weekly, the same eventual decrease in interferon inducibility has been seen as noted with other interferon inducers. This result will clearly be limiting if a constant blood level must be maintained in order to achieve clinical efficacy. It may be possible, however, to circumvent hyporesponsive-ness pharmacologically, for example, by treatment with certain prostaglandin fractions (Stringfellow, 1978). The most interesting biologic effects of poly ICLC to date have been seen in patients with myeloma and juvenile laryngeal papillomatosis, as reported previously in preliminary trials of purified human interferon (Einhorn and Strander, 1977; Mellstedt et al., 1979).

A large body of data generated with animal tumor models or with tissue culture systems, as well as an intuitive expectation, suggests that interferon (and inducers), if effective in cancer treatment, will be more so in patients with low tumor burdens treated early in the natural history of their disease than in patients with extensive, refractory disease. Further clinical trials of these putative biologic response modifiers should devolve about such patients. It remains to be seen whether the autochthonous tumors of man will demonstrate the wame clinically significant interferon response observed in transplantable rodent tumor systems of in rodent tumors known to be induced by virus (Gresser and Tovey, 1978).

The antitumor mechanism of poly ICLC (if it in fact exists) would undoubtedly be complex, involving all of the possibilities described for interferon per se, e.g., alterations in membrane structure and function, enhanced natural killer cell activity, increased expression of cell surface antigens, and altered macromolecular synthetic processes, as well as possible mechanisms related to the polynucleotide itself (Levy and Levine, 1982). Further clinical trials with poly ICLC are underway since induction of a diversity of interferon species can be postulated to represent an advantage over the administration of one species of molecularly cloned interferon.

REFERENCES

Beers, R.F., and Braun, W. 1971, in: Beers, R.F. and Braun W. eds.,
    "Biological Effects of Polynucleotides", p.3, Springer-Verlag,
    New York.
Buckler, C.E., Dubuy, H.G., Johnson, M.L. and Baron, S. 1971,
    Kinetics of serum interferon response in mice after single and
    multiple injections of poly I-poly C, Proc. Soc. Exp. Biol.
    Med., 136:394.
Catalano, L.W., and Baron, S. 1970, Protection against herpes virus
    and encephalomyocarditis virus encephalitis with a double-
    stranded RNA inducer of interferon, Proc. Soc. Exp. Biol. Med.,
    133:684.
Cone, E.R., and Johnson, A.G. 1971, Regulation of the immune system
    by synthetic polynucleotides. III. Action on antigen reactive
    cells of thymic origin, J. Exp. Med., 133:665.
Drake, W.P., Cimino, E.F., Mardiney, M.R., and Sutherland, J.C. 1974,
    Prophylactic therapy of spontaneous leukemia in AKR mice by
    polyadenylic-polyuridylic acid, J. Natl. Cancer Inst., 52:941.
DuBuy, H.G., Johnson, M.L., Buckler, C.E., and Baron, S. 1970,
    Relationship between dose size and dose interval of
    polyinosinic-polycytidyclic acid and interferon
    hyporesponsiveness in mice, Proc. Soc. Exp. Biol. Med, 135:340.
Einhorn, S., and Strander, H. 1977, in: Stinebring, R. and Chapple,
    P., eds. "Human Interferon Production and Clinical Use", Plenum
    Press, New York.
Field, A.J., Tytell, A.A., Lampson, G.P., and Hilleman, M.R. 1967,
    Inducers of interferon and host resistance. II. Multistranded
    synthetic polynucleotide complexes, Proc. Natl. Acad. Sci., USA,
    58:1004.
Field, A.K., Tytell, A.A., Piperno, E., Lampson, G.P. Nemes, M.M.,
    and Hilleman, M.R. 1972, Poly I:C: an inducer of interferon and
    interference against virus infection, Medicine (Baltimore),
    51:169.
Finter, N.B. 1973, Interferon and inducers in vivo: I. Antiviral
    effects in experimental animals in: Finter, N.B. ed.,
    "Interferons and Interferon Inducers", Amsterdam: North Holland
    Publishing Co., pp. 295-361.
Glasgow, L.A., Crane, J.L., Jr., and Kern, E.R. 1978, Antitumor
    activity of interferon against murine osteogenic sarcoma cells
    in vitro, J. Natl. Cancer Inst., 60:659.
Greenberg, L.A., Pollard, R.B., Lutwick, L.I., Gregory, P.B.,
    Robinson, W.S., and Merigan, T.C., 1976, Effect of human
    leukocyte interferon on hepatitis B virus infection in patients
    with chronic active hepatitis, N. Engl. J. Med., 295:517.
Gresser, I. 1977, Antitumor effects of interferon in: Becker, R.,
    ed. "Cancer - A Comprehensive Treatise". Plenum Press, New York,
    5:521.
Gresser, I., Maury, C., Bandu, M.T., Tovey, M., and Maunoury, M.T.
    1978, Role of endogenous interferon in the anti-tumor effect of
    poly I-C and statolon as demonstrated by the use of anti-mouse
    interferon serum, Int. J. Cancer, 21:72.

Gresser, I., and Tovey, M.G. 1978, Biochim. Biophys. Acta., 516:231.

Hill, N.O., Loeb, E., Pardue, A., Dorn, G.L., Khan, A., and Hill, J.M. 1979, J. Clin. Hematol. Oncol., 9:137.

Hilleman, M.R. 1968, Interferon induction and Utilization, J. Cell Physiol., 71:43.

Ho, M., and Armstrong, J.A. 1975, Interferon, Ann. Rev. Micro., 29:131.

Kern, R.R., Overall, J.C., and Glasgow, L.A. 1975, Herpes virus hominis infection in newborn mice: Treatment with the interferon inducer polyinosinic-polycytidylic acid, Antimicrob Agents Chemother., 7:793.

Kreider, J.W., and Benjamin, S.A. 1972, Tumor immunity and the mechanism of polyinosinic-polycytidylic acid inhibition of tumor growth, J. Natl. Cancer Inst., 49:1303.

Krown, S.E., Kerr, D., Stewart, W.E., Pollack, M.S., Cunningham-Rundles, S., Hirshaut, Y., Pinsky, C.M., Levy, H.B., and Oettgen, H.F. 1981, Phase I Trial of Poly ICLC in Patients with Advanced Cancer in: "Augmenting Agents in Cancer Therapy", (Hersh, E.M., Chirigos, M.A., and Mastrangelo, M.J., eds.) Raven Press, pp. 165-176.

Lacour, F., Delage, G., and Chianale, C. 1975, Reduced incidence of spontaneous mammary tumors in C3H/He mice after treatment with polyadenylate-polyuridylate, Science, 187:256.

Lacour, F., Delage, G., Spira, A., Nahon-Merlin, E., Lacour, J., Michaelson, A.M., and Bayet, S. 1982a, Randomized trial with poly A-poly U as adjuvant therapy complimenting surgery in patients with breast cancer: In vitro studies of cellular immunity. n: "Recent Results in Cancer Research", Bonnadonna, G., Mathe, G., and Salmon, S.E., eds., Springer-Verlag, Berlin.

Lacour, F., Lacour, J., Spira, A., Michaelson, A.M., Delage, G., Petit, J.Y., and Viguier, J. 1982b, A new adjuvant treatment with polyadenylic-polyuridylic acid in operable breast cancer. In: "Recent Results in Cancer Research", Mathe, G., Bonnadonna, G., and Salmon, S.E. eds., Springer-Verlag, Berlin.

Lacour, F., Spira, A., Lacour, J., and Prade, M. 1972, Polyadenylic-polyuridylic acid, an adjunct to surgery in the treatment of spontaneous mammary tumours in C3H/He mice and transplantable melanoma in the hamster, Cancer Res., 32:648.

Lampkin, B.C., Levine, A.S., Levy, H.B., Krivit, W.A., and Hammond, D. 1982, Phase II Trial of Poly (ICLC) (An Interferon Inducer) in the Treatment of Children with Acute Leukemia. Proceedings of the American Society of Clinical Oncology (Abstract C-476).

Leventhal, B.G., Kashima, H., Levine, A.S. and Levy, H.B. 1981, Treatment of Recurrent Laryngeal Papillomatosis with an Artificial Interferon Inducer (Poly ICLC), J. Pediatrics, 99:614.

Levine, A.S., Durie, B., Lampkin, B., Leventhal, B.G., and Levy, H.B. 1981, Poly (ICLC): Interferon Induction, Toxicity, and Clinical Efficacy in Leukemia, Lymphoma, Solid Tumors, Myeloma, and Laryngeal Papillomatosis. In "Augmenting Agents in Cancer Therapy", (E.M. Hersh, et al., ed.) Raven Press, 151.

Levine, A.S., Durie, B., Lampkin, B., Leventhal, B.G., and Levy, H.B.
    1982, Interferon Induction, Toxicity, and Clinical Efficacy of
    Poly ICLC in Hematologic Malignancies and Other tumors in:
    "Immunotherapy of Human Cancer" (W. Terry and S. Rosenberg,
    eds.) Elsevier North Holland, Inc., 411.
Levine, A.S., Sivulich, M., Wiernick, P.H., and Levy, H.B. 1979,
    Initial clinical trials in cancer patients of polyriboinosinic-
    polyribocytidylic acid stabilized with poly-1-lysine, in
    carboxymethylcellulose [Poly (ICLC)[, a highly effective
    interferon inducer, Cancer Res., 39:1645.
Levy, H.B. 1977, Induction of interferon in vivo by polynucleotides,
    Tex. Rep. Biol. Med., 35:91.
Levy, H.B., Asofsky, R., and Riley, R. 1970, The mechanism of the
    antitumor action of poly I-poly C, Ann. N.Y. Acad. Sci.,
    173:640.
Levy, H.B., Baer, G., Baron, S., Buckler, C.E., Gibbs, C.J.,
    Iadarola, M.J., London, W.T., and Rice, J.A. 1975, A modified
    polyriboninosinic-polyribocytidylic acid complex that induces
    interferon in primates, Infect. Dis., 132:434.
Levy, H.B., and Levine, A.S. 1982, Antitumor effects of interferon
    and poly ICLC, and their possible utility as anti-neoplastic
    agents in man, Texas Repts. Biol. and Med., in press.
Levy, H.B., London, W., Fuccillo, D.A., Baron, S. and Rice, J. 1976,
    Prophylactic control of simian hemorrhagic fever in monkeys by
    an interferon inducer, polyriboinosinic-polyribocytidylic
    acid-poly-L-lysine, Infect. Disease, 133:A256.
Mellstedt, H., Ahre, A., Bjorkholm, M. et al. 1979, Interferon
    therapy in myelomatosis, Lancet, 1:245.
Merigan, T.C., Sikora, K., Breeden, J.H. et al. 1978, Preliminary
    observations on the effects of interferon in non-Hodgkin's
    lymphoma, N. Engl. J. Med., 299:1449.
Merigan, T.C., and Regelson, W. 1967, Interferon induction in man by
    a synthetic polyanion of defined composition, N. Eng. J. Med.,
    277:1283.
Morahan, P., Barnes, D., and Munson, A. 1978, Relationship of
    molecular weight to antiviral and antitumor activities and toxic
    effects of maleic anhydride - divinyl either (MVE) polyanions,
    Cancer Treat. Rep., 62:1797.
Niblack, J.F. 1977, Studies with low molecular weight inducers of
    interferon in man, Tex. Rep. Bio. Med, 35:528.
Nordlund, J., Wolff, S., and Levy, H.B. 1970, Inhibition of
    biological activity of polyinosinic-polycytidylic acid by human
    plasma, Proc. Soc. Exp. Biol. Med., 133:439.
Oie, H.K., Buckler, C.E., Uhlendorf, C.P., Hill, D., and Baron, S.
    1972, Improved assays for a variety of interferons, Proc. Soc.
    Exp. Biol. Med., 140:1178.
Pavilides, N., Schultz, R., Chirigos, M., and Leutzeler, J. 1978,
    Effect of maleic anhydride-divinyl ether copolymers on
    experimental M109 metastases and macrophage tumoricidal
    function, Cancer Treat. Rep., 62:1817.

Purcell, R.H., London, W.T., McAuliffe, V.J. et al., 1976, Modification of chronic hepatitis-B virus infection in chimpanzees by administration of an interferon inducer, Lancet, 1:757.

Regelson, W. 1976, Clinical immunoadjuvant studies with tilorone DEAA Fluorene (RMI 11002DA) and Corynebacterium Parvum, and some observations on the role of host resistance and herpes-like lesions in tumor growth, Ann. N.Y. Acad. Sci., 277:269.

Robinson, R.A., DeVita, V.T., Levy, H.B., Baron, S., Hubbard, S.P., and Levine, A.S. 1976, A Phase I-II trial of multiple-dose polyribinosinic-polyribocytidylic acid in patients with leukemia or solid tumors, J. Natl. Cancer Inst., 57:599.

Sarma, P.S., Shiu, G., Neubauer, R., Baron, S., and Huebner, R. 1969, Virus induced sarcoma of mice. Inhibition by a synthetic polyribonucleotide complex, Proc. Natl. Acad. Sci., USA, 62:1146.

Scheid, M.D., Hoffman, M.K., Kumuro, D., Hammerling, O., Abbot, J., Boyse, E.A., Cohen, G.H., Hooper, J.A., Schulof, R.S., and Goldstein, A.L. 1973, Differentiation of T cells induced by preparations from thymic and non-thymic agents, J. Exp. Med., 138:1027.

Schmidtke, J.R., and Johnson, A.G. 1971, Regulation of the immune system by synthetic polynucleotides. I. Characteristics of adjuvant action on antibody synthesis, J. Immunol., 106:1191.

Skurkivich, S.V., Makhonova, L.A., Mayakova, S.A., Arkhipova, N.A., Olshanskaya, N.V., Sikorova, S.N., Kogan, E.M., Tomkovsky, A., Bresler, S., Gavrilova, E.A., and Krokhina, M.A. 1977, Interferon therapy of an acute leukemia patient in: "Interferon Scientific Memoranda (Memo 1-A410)" Calspan Corporation, Buffalo, New York.

Steinberg, A.D., Baron, S., and Talal, N. 1969, The pathogenesis of autoimmunity in New Zealand mice. I. Induction of antinucleic acid antibodies by polyinosinic-polycytidylic acid, Proc. Natl. Acad. Sci., USA, 63:1102.

Stolfi, R., and Martin, D. 1978, Therapeutic activity of maleic anhydride-vinylether compounds against spontaneous autochthonous murine mammary tumors, Cancer Treat. Rep., 62:1791.

Stringfellow, D.A. 1980, Interferon Induction: Theory and Experimental Application. In: "Interferon and Interferon Inducers" (Stringfellow, D.A., ed.) pp. 145-165, New York: Marcel Dekker, Inc.

Stringfellow, D.A. 1978, Prostaglandin restoration of the interferon response in hyporeactive animals, Science, 201:376.

Wampler, G.L., Kuperminc, M., and Regelson, W. 1973, Phase I study of tilorone, a non-marrow depressing antitumor agent, Cancer Chemo. Rep., 57:209.

Wanebo, H.Y., Kemeny, M., Pinsky, C.M., Hirshaut, Y., and Oettgen, H.F. 1976, Infleunce of poly A-poly on immune response of cancer patients, Ann. N.Y. Acad. Sci., 277:288.

Zeleznick, C.D., and Bhuyan, B.K. 1969, Treatment of leukemic (L-1210) mice with double-stranded polyribonucleotides, Proc. Soc. Exp. Biol. Med., 130:126.

TOXICITY OF INTERFERON

HOWARD M. SMEDLEY AND TERENCE WHEELER

Ludwig Institute for Cancer Research, MRC Centre
Hills Road, Cambridge and Department of Radiotherapy
Addenbrooke's Hospital, Hills Road, Cambridge

INTRODUCTION

Shortly after their discovery, interferons were found to have anti-viral and anti-proliferative activity. This led to the hope that they might have some role as therapeutic agents in the treatment of viral and neoplastic diseases. Early in vitro and in vivo work suggested that interferon was capable of causing lysis and death of cells in culture media (Nissen et al., 1977). Further in vivo testing in experimental animal systems soon showed that interferons exhibit a species specificity for both therapeutic and toxic effects (Gresser et al., 1981). In consequence, animal models (including primates) have not been capable of demonstrating all the toxicities exhibited when interferons have been used in human subjects. In addition, as different species of interferon have been isolated and purified for human use, it is becoming apparent that each specific type may have a different spectrum of activities and this includes unwanted toxic effects. It is therefore impossible to extrapolate from experience with one interferon to the effects of another interferon, even in similar clinical circumstances. It is also not yet known what effect, if any, the particular disease being treated has on the host response and susceptibility to the effects of interferon. This chapter aims to review some of the toxicities which appear to be common to all series so far reported and then to discuss in some detail the experience of one group using highly purified DNA recombinant interferon in advanced malignancy.

CLINICAL EXPERIENCE

The limiting factor in most series treating patients with interferon has been the quantity and purity of the preparations

available. This has inevitably meant that experience is limited and
most series contain less than 20 patients. The first reported series
used interferons with a purity of the order of 1%, using doses of 3 x
10^6 i.u. by intramuscular injection daily initially followed by
reduction to 3 x 10^6 i.u. three times per week for patients whose
disease exhibited some response. Early clinical experience suggested
that interferon administration was associated with rapid onset of
fever and shivering and that a significant number of patients
experienced pain at the site of injection together with general
malaise and frequent headaches. It was not possible to determine in
these early studies whether the toxicity observed was an intrinsic
property of the interferons used or a consequence of pyrogenic
impurities present in the injected solution. Several experiments
were designed to answer this question. Finter et al. (1982)
published results of an experiment in which Patas monkeys were dosed
daily for 15 days with 2 x 10^6 i.u./kg body weight using lymphoblastoid human interferon (Namalwa line) with a specific activity of
2 x 10^7 i.u./mg protein. They found no changes in rectal temperature
or peripheral white blood counts and similar results were obtained
when rhesus monkeys were used as the model system. They concluded
that toxicities reported from other studies using less purified
material may well have been caused by inadvertent contamination. It
was stressed that their animal data could not be extrapolated to man.
In a further study, Scott et al. (1981) published the results of
toxicity studies using healthy, fit human volunteers. Partially
purified interferon (PIF) at a purity of 1.5 x 10^6 i.u. per mg of
protein was compared against interferon purified by passage through a
monoclonal antibody affinity chroma- tography column with a resultant
activity of 100 x 10^6 i.u. per mg of protein. After intramuscular
injection both interferons caused tachycardia and pyrexia, general
malaise and headache. Although slightly lower peak serum levels of
the highly purified interferon were found in the patients, no
difference was found between the two groups on objective scoring of
signs and symptoms. The authors therefore concluded that the
purification of interferon has no effect on its toxicity which must
be considered as an intrinsic property of the interferon, or at least
of the preparation studied. More recent experience with very highly
purified recombinant DNA interferons in adequate numbers of patients
has confirmed these suspicions.

Pyrexia

Pyrexia with rectal temperatures of over 38°C are found in all
patients after injection of doses of interferon commonly encountered
in clinical practice (greater than one million units). This change
is seen within three hours of administration of the interferon and
does not appear to be dose related. Temperature will spontaneously
subside from 12 to 24 hr and in patients receiving regular daily
doses of interferon, tachyphylaxis will develop after approximately
two weeks of therapy. Pyrexia may be prevented by prophylactic

administration of paracetamol 600 mg by mouth one hour prior to
injection of interferon.

Headache and Myalgia

These symptoms are reported in the majority of patients
receiving interferon in therapeutic doses. They most frequently
appear on the first day of treatment, some eight to 12 hr following
injection, and can recur following each daily dose. They also appear
to be independent of the dose and tachyphylaxis has also commonly
been observed. Paracetamol again appears to be effective in
controlling these symptoms.

Fatigue

Many patients complain of fatigue, which characteristically
occurs between four and seven days after initiation of therapy. The
severity and duration of fatigue appears to be dose related, being
more severe at higher dose levels, although in all cases it is found
to be reversible. Patients becoming extremely lethargic and
unwilling to take food or drink are in danger of exacerbating a
catabolic state and it is for this reason that fatigue may be a
serious and unacceptable side effect for cancer patients who are
already be cachectic and nutritionally compromised. Some investigators have found that fatigue is a dose limiting toxicity in
clinical studies.

Gastrointestinal Symptoms

Anorexia and nausea may occur early in the clinical course of
treatment and are often associated with malaise and fatigue. They
occur approximately three days after starting treatment and are dose
related. Both symptoms add significantly to the problems of managing
patients with cancer. Patients who are warned of the likelihood of
anorexia and provided with dietetic advice often tolerate treatment
better than patients not advised in this manner. Weight loss is
common in patients having interferon therapy and is almost certainly
a consequence of anorexia and fatigue. Diarrhoea has been described
in approximately 25% of patients having treatment during the first
two weeks of therapy and the mechanism is unclear. Some association
with altered dietary intake cannot be excluded.

Nervous System

Transient paraesthesia, particularly in the fingers, is
recognized in approximately 10% of patients receiving interferon
therapy. Again, this has been used as a signal to stop interferon
therapy by some investigators. However, in those patients in whom
high dose therapy was continued further neurological signs have been
observed, mainly weakness, confusion, dysarthria and loss of short-

term memory. All these symptoms are reversible on stopping therapy
and it is interesting to speculate that the fatigue, noted by all
investigators at low doses of interferon, may represent one end of a
spectrum of interferon effects on the central nervous system. The
mechanism of action on the CNS is unknown. Interferon is not found
in the cerebral spinal fluid of animals or patients when doses of up
to 20×10^6 i.u. are administered i.m. and thus is not thought to
cross the blood brain barrier. The clinical findings of reversible
CNS toxicity with high dose interferon are of potential importance
because they may represent a dose limiting toxicity. The mechanism
for these effects cannot be explained as yet.

Peripheral Blood Count

     Falls in the level of the circulating leukocytes in the
peripheral blood have been reported in most interferon studies.
Falls from the normal level are commonly detected 24 hr after
starting therapy. There have been no reported cases of irreversible
leukopenia and in all reported series leukopenia is transient and
rarely causes the white count to fall below 2000 cells/ml of blood.
No cases of septicemia or opportunistic infection have been
attributed to interferon. It has been suggested that the degree of
leukopenia may be related to the therapeutic value for any individual
patient. Transient falls in platelet count have also been commonly
observed following the same time scale as the leukocyte count. There
is no reported case of the platelet count falling below 100,000/ml.
Hemoglobin levels are not significantly affected by the administration of interferon.

Hepatic Enzyme Abnormalities

     Measurments of liver function tests in patients undergoing
interferon treatment have shown no consistent alteration in serum
bilirubin or alkaline phosphatase levels. However the serum transaminases, e.g. S.G.P.T. and S.G.O.T., frequently show elevation,
often to four times normal serum levels. Although this has been used
to limit dosage given in Phase I studies there are no reported cases
in the literature of permanent hepatic damage resulting from
interferon therapy and many observers report enzyme levels returning
to normal spotaneously some three to four weeks after initiation of
therapy without altering the dose. Explanation for these biochemical
changes is unclear but it is interesting to note that several
investigators used this parameter to determine the quantity of
interferon administered to patients in Phase I studies. This may
explain why there is some discrepancy in descriptions of toxicities
observed by investigators who have continued treatment despite rising
levels of SGPT and have therefore given their patients greater
amounts of interferon and have observed different dose limiting
toxicities after greater duration of therapy.

THE CAMBRIDGE BREAST TRIAL

   Recombinant DNA technology has made it possible to prepare
interferons of high purity in sufficient quantities to allow proper
prospective clinical trials to take place. This will allow
sufficient numbers of patients to be studied to answer many of the
questions relating to the intrinsic toxicities and therapeutic
benefits of the interferons. In Cambridge patients with locally
advanced breast cancer which has failed to respond to all modalities
of conventional therapy (surgery, radiation, hormonal and cytotoxic
regimes) are being treated with human leukocyte A interferon of
greater than 96% purity (Hoffmann–La Roche). Patients entered for
the trial have some form of disease which is assessable to objective
measurement, although visceral metastases may also be present. The
aim of the study is to determine the safety and efficacy of
interferon in advanced breast cancer. Patients are allocated to one
of two arms, the first group receive a daily intra–muscular injection
of rIFLαA at a dose of 20×10^6 units per m^2. The second group
receive intra–muscular injectiosn three times per week at a dose of
50 million units per m^2. The aim is to continue treatment for 12
weeks, at which point the patient is fully re–asessed and treatment
may then be discontinued or, in patients showing objective response
to disease, may be continued with a maintenance regime. At time of
writing 12 patients have completed therapy and although it is
premature to present response data, a predictable pattern of toxicity
has emerged in all our patients and which has caused us to develop a
supportive care program to minimize and treat these symptoms whilst
being able to maintain high dose levels of therapy. Table I outlines
the profile of toxicities experienced in the first patients treated
with rIFLαA.

   At these doses, seven of the patients developed chronic lethargy
and somnolence by the third week of treatment causing them to spend
up to 20 hr per day asleep and consequently unable to take any form
of nourishment. This resulted in significant weight loss. Five
patients developed frank confusion, loss of concentration and
expressive dysphasia. Two patients developed peripheral parasthesia
and one patient developed upper motor neurone lesion signs in the
lower limbs. All patients returned to normal within seven – ten days
of withdrawal of interferon and have subsequently tolerated the
re–introduction of interferon therapy at a reduced dose. Four
patients have died whilst on therapy and while death can unequivo-
cally ascribed to advanced disease in two patients, it is possible
that in the remaining two the patients extreme lethargy and
consequent dehydration was a contributory factor to death. Investigation of the first patient to develop these effects revealed no
evidence of intracranial metastases to account for the symptoms. An
EEG taken during the confusional state showed a grossly abnormal
pattern with excess slow wave activity. No base line EEG had been
taken on this patient for comparison. However, base line EEG's have

TABLE I

Side Effects of rIFL–αA in 10 Patients

	Time of Onset After Start of Treatment	Duration	No. of Patients Affected	Dose Related
Pyrexia	1 hr	2– 3 days	10	No
Myalgia	2– 3 days	4– 7 days	10	No
Nausea & Vomiting	2– 3 days	7–10 days	10	Yes
Headache	2– 3 days	7–14 days	4	Yes
Neuropathy	7 days	7–10 days	3	Yes
Lethargy	7–10 days	3– 4 weeks	10	Yes
Anorexia & Weight Loss	10–14 days	3– 4 weeks	8	Yes
C.N.S. Toxicity	21–28 days	7–14 days	2	Yes

been obtained in all subsequent patients admitted to the study, which, without exception, have been normal. Subsequent EEG's obtained at four, 12 and 14 weeks have shown a consistent abnormality of generalized increase in slow wave activity with one patient developing electrophysiological features in keeping with early encephalopathy (Fig. 1). Repeat EEG's after withdrawal of therapy showed return to normal activity. All patients exhibiting symptoms of CNS toxicity have been investigated to exclude intracranial metastases and in no patient has cerebral metastases been discovered either during life or at post mortem. Similar CNS toxicity manifested as drowsiness and disorientation has been reported (Rohatiner, 1983) in patients receiving IFN–α 100 x 10^6 units/m^2 daily for seven days in the treatment of hematological malignancies. They also reported reversible EEG abnormalities with increasing diffuse slow wave activity and decreased attenuation on eye opening. This distressing clinical syndrome is naturally cause for cessation of therapy and consequently should be avoided wherever possible. In our experience this is best achieved by reducing interferon dose to 50% of the original dose at the first sign of profound lethargy and any suggestion of serious and continuing weight loss. It is interesting

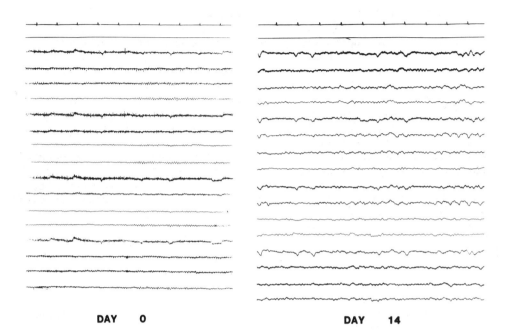

DAY   0   **DAY   14**

Fig. 1. EEG's from 62 year old patient with breast carcinoma prior
to and 14 days into Hu rIFNαA administration (36 x 10 units
daily).

to note that this side effect was not reported in Phase I studies of
the same preparation. A likely explanation for this is that the
investigators in these studies also noted fatigue and drowsiness but
stopped administration of interferon when the serum transaminases
rose beyond a certain level. In our experience this biochemical
toxicity is manifest some seven to ten days before the onset of
severe CNS effects.

TREATMENT OF TOXICITY

Patients undergoing unpleasant cytotoxic chemotherapy are known
to tolerate such treatment better if treatment is explained to them
by their physician and they understand the need to accept such
therapy. The same is true of interferon treatment and we believe
patients undergoing such therapy should be fully informed about the
nature of their disease and the treatment proposed. In our study all
treatments are administered by the same team each day and this allows
a rapport to develop between patient and staff. Prior to the first
injection patients are given paracetamol, 1 gm orally 60 minutes
prior to injection. They then receive 3 g of paracetamol daily in
divided doses for the first four to six days of treatment, after

which time paracetamol is given as required. Patients also have an
interview with a dietician who advises about diets likely to be
suitable for the individual patient during the period of profound
anorexia. Dietary supplements in the form of high calorie liquids
are also provided and the patient encouraged to have a defined
calorific intake. The patient living alone should be admitted to a
hostel in order that nursing supervision can be given for the first
two to three weeks of therapy. Nausea has been controlled with pro-
chloperazine 5 mg by mouth t.d.s. but occasionally this may by
administered in the form of suppositories. If a patient shows
evidence of unduly marked lethargy and drowsiness after one week of
therapy the dose of interferon is reduced to 50% dose level until the
patient shows signs of recovery and returns to base line activity.
We believe that with prompt recognition of toxicity and appropriate
reduction in dose it should be possible to maintain all patients on
interferon therapy without undue and unacceptable toxicity.

REFERENCES

Finter, N.B., Woodroffe, J., and Priestman, T.J. 1982, Monkeys are
     insensitive to pyrogenic effects of human alpha-interferons,
     Nature, 298:301.
Gresser, I., Aguet, M., Morel-Maroger, L., Woodrow, D., Puvion-
     Dutillel, F., Guillon, J., and Maury, C. 1981, Electro-
     phorectically pure mouse interferon inhibits growth, induces
     liver and kidney lesions, and kills suckling mice, American
     Journal of Pathology, 102:396.
Nissen, C., Speck, B., Emödi, G., and Iscove, N.N. 1977, Toxicity of
     human leucocyte interferon preparations in human bone-marrow
     cultures, The Lancet, 1:203.
Rohatiner, A., Prior, P., Burton, A.L., Smith, A.T., Balkwill, F.R.,
     and Lister, T.A. CNS toxicity of interferon, Br. J. Cancer, in
     press.
Scott, G.M., Secher, D.S., Flowers, D., Bate, J., Cantell, K., and
     Tyrrell, D. 1981, Toxicity of interferon, Brit. Med. J.,
     282:1345.

CONTRIBUTORS

ERNEST C. BORDEN, University of Wisconsin Clinical Cancer Center, Madison

LARS-ÅKE BROSTRÖM, Department of Orthopaedic Surgery, Karolinska Hospital, Stockholm, Sweden

W. COURTNEY McGREGOR, Biopolymer Research Department, Hoffmann-La Roche Inc., Nutley, New Jersey

THOMAS L. DAO, Rosewell Park Memorial Institute, Buffalo

ZOFIA E. DZIEWANOWSKA, Department of Medical Oncology and Immunology, Central Research Division, Hoffmann-La Roche Inc., Nutley, New Jersey

ION GRESSER, Institut de Recherches Scientifiques sur le Cancer, Villejuif, France

JORDAN U. GUTTERMAN, M.D. Anderson Hospitals and Tumor Institute, Houston

KIMIYOSHI HIRAKAWA, Department of Microbiology, Kyoto Prefectural University of Medicine, Japan

JAMES F. HOLLAND, Mount Sinai Hospital and School of Medicine, New York

LARS R. HOLSTI, Department of Radiotherapy and Oncology, Helsinki University Central Hospital, Helsinki, Finland

SANDRA HORNING, Department of Medicine, Division of Oncology, Stanford University Medical Center, Stanford

DRAGO IKIĆ, Center for Research and Standardization of Immunologic Substances, Department of Medical Sciences, Yugoslav Academy of Sciences and Arts, Zagreb, Yugoslavia

TSUNATARO KISHIDA, Department of Neurosurgery, Kyoto Prefectural University of Medicine, Japan

211

ARTHUR S. LEVINE, Division of Cancer Treatment, National Cancer
    Institute, Bethesda, Maryland

KARIN MATTSON, Department of Pulmonary Disease, Helsinki University
    Central Hospital, Helsinki, Finland

YOSHIO NAKAGAWA, Department of Microbiology, Kyoto Prefectural
    University of Medicine, Japan

JOHN R. NEEFE, Divisions of Medical Oncology and Immunologic Oncology,
    Lombardi Cancer Research Center and Department of Medicine,
    Georgetown University, Washington, D.C.

ULF NILSONNE, Department of Orthopaedic Surgery, Karolinska Hospital,
    Stockholm, Sweden

TERENCE J. PRIESTMAN, Department of Radiotherapy and Oncology, Queen
    Elizabeth and Duley Road Hospitals, Birmingham

ARMIN H. RAMEL, Biopolymer Research Department, Hoffmann–La Roche
    Inc., Nutley, New Jersey

AMA ROHATINER, I.C.R.F. Department of Medical Oncology, St.
    Bartholomew's Hospital, London

GEOFFREY M. SCOTT, Clinical Research Centre, Harrow, Middlesex

STEPHEN A. SHERWIN, Division of Cancer Treatment, National Cancer
    Institute, Bethesda, Maryland

KAROL SIKORA, Ludwig Institute for Cancer Research, Cambridge

HOWARD M. SMEDLEY, Ludwig Institute for Cancer Research, Cambridge

KENZO SUZUKI, Department of Microbiology, Kyoto Prefectural University
    of Medicine, Japan

SATOSHI UEDA, Department of Neurosurgery, Kyoto Prefectural University
    of Medicine, Japan

DAVID TYRRELL, Division of Communicable Disease, Clinical Research
    Centre, Harrow

ANNAPURNA VYAKARNAM, Ludwig Institute for Cancer Research, Cambridge

TERENCE K. WHEELER, Department of Radiotherapy, Addenbrooke's
    Hospital, Cambridge

BRYAN R.G. WILLIAMS, Division of Infectious Diseases, Department of
    Paediatrics, The Hospital for Sick Children, Toronto

INDEX

213